BEAT
THE
FLU

BEAT
THE FLU

How to Stay Healthy through
the Coming Bird Flu Pandemic

A A Avlicino

Foreword by Dr Mike Skinner

To Enza & Poobear,
the only two women who have stood by me through my life.

Disclaimer

This book is for information purposes only. The author makes all the suggestions in this book in good faith. It is not intended to take the place of individual medical advice from a trained medical professional. Readers are advised to consult a doctor or other qualified health professional regarding treatment before acting on any information in this book, and it is up to the individual to exercise common sense and caution in implementing the author's recommendations in line with their own particular circumstances. To the best of the author's knowledge the information is correct at the time of going to press. The author, publisher and their employees or agents cannot accept responsibility for loss or damage suffered by individuals as a result of following advice within this book.

First published in 2006 by Fusion Press,
a division of Satin Publications Ltd.
101 Southwark Street
London SE1 0JF
UK
info@visionpaperbacks.co.uk
www.visionpaperbacks.co.uk
Publisher: Sheena Dewan

A catalogue record for this book is available from the British Library.

ISBN: 1-904132-87-1

2 4 6 8 10 9 7 5 3 1

Cover and text design by ok?design
Printed and bound in the UK by Mackays of Chatham Ltd, Chatham, Kent

Contents

Foreword by Dr Mike Skinner
BSc, PhD

It is a common accusation against scientists (particularly microbiologists) that we stir up fears to increase levels of funding. Those of us around in the mid to late 1980s will well remember the Government's AIDS broadcasts. I recollect how well those images of crumbling cliffs engendered an atmosphere of threat. There were tabloid reports criticising the campaign as scaremongering on the part of scientists and government officials. Where were the high numbers of cases? Wasn't this just a ruse by the scientists involved to raise more research funds? With 40 million HIV-infected people worldwide to date, it would be a foolish editor who raised such criticism nowadays. To be sure, the Western world figures have remained fairly low, lower than we might reasonably have hoped, but the reason for this might just be that the advertising campaign did its job. The level of cases in Africa and the relentless rise in the number of cases in developing countries such as India and China, as well as in the former Soviet bloc, is a clear indicator to us of what might have been.

So what about the threat from influenza? To say much would pre-empt Al's writing. Suffice it to say that in the time between the US swine flu scare of the mid 1970s and the mid 1990s, it was mainly those scientists working directly on the influenza virus who took the issue seriously. Most of the rest of us, facing issues such as HIV, Lassa and Ebola, and busily embracing the marvellous new techniques of molecular biology and immunology, thought of influenza in terms of the relatively mild pandemics that arise every ten years or so. Few of us gave much thought to the major pandemics that arise every 40 or 50 years – a severe pandemic like the Spanish Flu of 1918, which killed up to 50 million, was considered almost mythological. All this changed in 1997.

Up until that point few thought that Avian Influenza per se could pose a threat to humans. We assumed that pandemic strains were generated by recombination of avian and human strains, probably in pigs. Avian Influenza strains had long been handled safely in laboratories around the world. Such laboratories were secure to prevent the viruses escaping and threatening poultry, but relatively few measures were taken to protect the workers themselves, an approach justified by a 'long history of safe use'. Developments in Hong Kong in 1997 showed us that some Avian Influenza strains, such as the current H5N1, could infect humans and could kill. Since then we have seen the spread of H5N1 throughout the poultry flocks of South-East Asia, with dozens of human infections and high mortality. Fears are well grounded that a virus will arise that is able to spread easily amongst humans. We don't know when it will happen. That it has not happened yet, at the time of writing, shows it must be a rare event requiring particular conditions. Nor do we know what the resulting virus will be like. It could turn out to be a damp squib, a runt among pandemic influenza strains. It might turn to be like conventional pandemic strains that occur every decade or so. However, the unusual features of H5N1 in its current state mean that we would be negligent not to plan for the possibility, even the probability, that the resulting pandemic virus might retain its high virulence.

What of Al's book? It is accessible and very readable; its explanation of H5N1 assumes no background in biology, chemistry or medicine. Important and complicated concepts in virology, immunology and epidemiology are presented in a digestible form, soundly reflecting our current understanding. You will learn how H5N1 spreads and how to reduce the chances that you will be its next target. Al is honest and realistic about the risks of various pandemic scenarios and the precautions, some controversial, which would be appropriate.

Some elements of this book, and many of the reports in the popular press, bring to mind those films of the post-apocalyptic genre, with a few survivors attempting to rescue some relic of civilisation. If H5N1 does strike, and is as severe as we fear it might be, many millions will die and the effects on society will be considerable, but even Al's estimate of mortality is only about 6 to 8 per cent of the population (one in 12 to 15), which really does not compare with those films. Moreover the pandemic would pass relatively quickly, so that, for those who survive, 'rebuilding' can take place rapidly. The effects on us individually and on society as a whole can be mitigated by facing up to the risks and by careful planning for the most realistic scenarios. I hope that this book will prove a useful tool to those who take the threat seriously.

Dr Mike Skinner studied microbiology at the University of Leeds, followed by bacterial genetics and biochemistry for his PhD at the University of Leicester. He moved into the molecular biology of viruses, with postdoctoral positions on Coronaviruses pre-SARS (Würzburg, Germany), Poliovirus (Leicester and Reading) and HIV (MRC-Laboratory of Molecular Biology, Cambridge), before joining the Institute for Animal Health (London) as group leader to work on Avian Poxviruses. Since then he has also worked on two emerging poultry pathogens that have spread worldwide: Avian leukosis virus J and 'very virulent' Infectious bursal disease virus. He is now Senior Lecturer and Vaccine Vector Group Leader at the Department of Virology, Imperial College School of Medicine, London. His scientific interests are virus-host interactions and vaccines.

CHAPTER 1

The Coming Global Pandemic

Time bomb

The pandemic time bomb may have been activated. We are powerless to stop it or even slow it down. All the science we can muster, all the money we can spend, all the technology at our disposal may be swamped by this tsunami of disease. It may ravage cities, bring powerful countries to their knees and become the single greatest killer in centuries. The numbers it might kill are so large they challenge our comprehension.

The only way to grasp the magnitude of this coming pandemic is to break the numbers down to groups we can more easily imagine: the crowd in a stadium, the audience in a theatre, the passengers on a jet. It's as if a fully loaded Boeing 747 just crashed. Then 13 seconds later another 747. In just over 13 seconds two full plane-loads of people have been killed in an unprecedented tragedy that headlines the international news and galvanises the world. And then, after 13 more seconds, another one has crashed, bringing the death toll to more than 1,200 in just about 30 seconds. How could this happen? Could these deaths have been prevented? While you ponder these questions another 747 has crashed. Four jumbo jet-loads of people have died and the first minute is not even quite up yet.

In the next minute over 2,000 more people die. And in the next minute more than 2,000 additional people are gone. A sold-out Drury Lane Theatre in London or La Scala in Milan, all dead in a single minute. Wealth, position, status or lack thereof are not factors in this inconceivable scourge that kills more people in 90 seconds than the September 11 terrorist attacks on the US. And the deaths continue at this unimaginable rate, the equivalent to a packed Old Trafford or a Hiroshima A-bomb every 30 minutes. More people are killed in two hours than the 26 December Indian Ocean Tsunami. Every 24 hours another Melbourne, Caracas, Athens or Chicago dies. In three weeks the entire civilian and military death toll of World War II is exceeded. According to Michael Osterholm, director of the University of Minnesota's Center for Infectious Disease Research and Policy, by the time this unthinkable wave of death abates after a few months, 360 million people would be dead, a number equal to every man, woman and child in the US and Canada combined.

Even the number of nuclear blasts expected in the Cold War's Mutually Assured Destruction fell significantly short of killing 360 million people. The Pentagon estimated that 3,000 nuclear warheads dropped on the US would result in 25 million casualties and a similar number in the Soviet Union.

This is not the work of some genocidal terrorist. There is no terrorist weapon that can come close to approaching this level of fatality. Death on this scale can only be achieved by the impact of a giant asteroid – or a microscopic ghoul. The latter case will leave our cities standing, but they will be empty and sullen. This is not a quick global devastation of fire and brimstone. It is a slow global devastation of blood and phlegm and pain.

The way this pandemic kills is terrifyingly grisly. Historical accounts tell of people who were perfectly healthy in the morning, sick by lunchtime, and choking to death by evening. A massive immune reaction causes lungs to bubble up with a liquid froth of bloody pus spume, which is coughed up as a bright red soup and soon begins oozing from all over the body. Projectile nosebleeds are triggered by the tremendous pressures building up from inside. As the lungs can no longer get oxygen, the victims turn grey-blue. Swollen, covered in blood and pus, literally exploding from the fluid that inexorably pours into the lungs and under the skin, they suffocate and finally, mercifully, their lives end and so does their suffering.

The impossibly efficient killer capable of such destruction is not some Dr Strangelove complex mechanical nuclear fission device but a microscopic clump of protein so small it would take a thousand placed end-to-end to stretch across the diameter of a human hair. Medieval philosophers were obsessed with how many angels could dance on the head of a pin. If we consider these tiny demons instead of the usual angels, the answer is that over 300 million can perform their dance of death on the head of that same pin.

This infinitesimal blob of organic matter that staggers the imagination is neither truly living nor inanimate. It is neither a single-celled nor a multicellular organism. It is a virus, a term that everyone has heard of but few people truly comprehend. It can best be described as a chunk of genetic material wrapped up in a protein shell, whose only reason for existence is to infect living cells, forcing them to make copies of the virus itself until they burst, the copies then repeating the same cycle themselves.

It's named in the medical vernacular: H5N1. A cryptic name for what may end up being the greatest killer of the century. H5N1 is a virus that medical authorities around the world are virtually unanimously claiming will be the source of the next human pandemic. Not just an epidemic, restricted to one unlucky geographical location, but a true pandemic, a runaway epidemic on a global scale. It has earned the title 'Bird Ebola' for the horrific and swift manner it kills its avian hosts by liquifying them from the inside. H5N1 has been primarily restricted to birds in Asia up until the time of this book going to press, and only a few dozen humans have died from it, therefore at first glance this virus hardly seems the primary candidate for any type of significant global scourge. Indeed, in its present form, it is unlikely to present any significant pandemic threat. The key phrase, however, is 'in its present form'.

H5N1 has been evolving before researchers' eyes. All evidence points to the fact that this virus will soon hybridise itself into a form that can be spread from person to person as easily as a common cold. It is virtually inevitable. In that case, it is only a matter of time until H5N1 may go on to infect thousands, then millions, then billions of people. Of those it infects, it may kill one out of ten, or maybe as many as one out of three. And there is absolutely nothing that anyone can do to stop it.

There is barely enough antiviral in the world today to help less than one in a thousand people survive. There is no vaccine known to be effective, and there may not be. There is no treatment.

No one can know the future and no one can predict what form the continuing evolution of the H5N1 virus will take. It may continue in its inexorable march towards a human pandemic or at any given time it might

The Coming Global Pandemic

take an evolutionary left turn and recombine with some unrelated animal virus and end up being a plague only for pigs, voles, koalas or some other animal. However, I'm not willing to bet my life on the chance that the evolutionary direction of this unpredictable ball of protein is going to only target fuzzy marsupials munching on eucalyptus leaves. There are steps that you can take right now to increase the chance that you and your loved ones will survive.

It will take significant effort, perseverance and forethought on your part. If you adopt the attitude 'it can't happen to me', it will be too late. If you think this is just more 'crying wolf' hype, it will be too late. If you wait until the pandemic is swamping your country and your medical system crumbles, it will be too late. By then, governments will be implementing arbitrary Draconian rules as to who will live and who will die. No country in the world has made arrangements for providing potentially life-saving preventative courses of antiviral to more than 3 per cent of its population. Many major developed countries have not even stockpiled enough preventative courses for a tiny fraction of 1 per cent of their people. It simply cannot be produced any faster. However, governmental myopia is also a significant factor even in light of the baleful statements that are being issued by leading authorities around the world:

This is a bomb that will impact the world.
Tommy Thompson, Former Secretary,
US Health and Human Services

[The H5N1 pandemic] is an absolute certainty.
Mike Leavitt, Secretary, US Health and Human Services

The number of people infected will go beyond billions because between 25 and 30% will fall ill.
Klaus Stohr, Director, WHO Global Influenza Center

This is a very ominous situation for the globe. It is the most important threat that we are facing right now.
Julie Gerberding, US Centers For Disease Control and Prevention

We don't know what the fatality will be but we can expect it to be very high. There will be enormous economic dislocation. Stock markets will close, international travel and trade will be limited.
Peter Cordingley, WHO regional spokesman

The best we can do is try to survive it. We need a Manhattan Project yesterday.
Paul Gully, Deputy Chief Public Health Officer, Canada

Short of thermonuclear war, I have a hard time imagining anything in my lifetime that would be as horrible.
Laurie Garrett, US Council on Foreign Relations Senior Fellow for Global Health

We're dealing here with world survival issues – or the survival of the world as we know it.
David Nabarro, United Nations Senior System Coordinator for Avian and Human Influenza

There is no 'magic bullet' against H5N1. Many of the world's best scientists have been trying to devise some way to counter or deflect this pandemic and so far have not succeeded. The majority of people on Earth are likely to be left unprotected and helpless against the wrath of this modern plague. If you want to do everything possible to help stay safe during this potential global illness, you must act now. Only then will you stand a good chance of letting this grim reaper pass you and your family by.

CHAPTER 2

What is H5N1?

Crossing the barrier of life

Viruses are formed of carbon-containing molecules that
have bizarrely evolved to self-assemble. To start with, we
have molecules that are nothing more than a collection of
atoms all strung together. We have all seen images of
models of molecules that look like billiard balls linked to
each other by small sticks. In the next moment we have
some of these molecules attaching themselves to specific
parts of the molecules nearby, making even more complex
molecules.

So far so good. We know that molecules have particular
points on their structures that attract other molecules in a
virtually magnetic fashion. That's an important factor;
otherwise, living beings like us that are built up of complex
carbon-containing molecules wouldn't exist. However,
these assemblages of carbon, oxygen, hydrogen and other
atoms come together in very specific sequences. Molecule
A fits into Molecule B, which combines with Molecule C,
which hooks up with Molecule D, and pretty soon we
have a virus.

Viruses don't fit the textbook definition of life as they
can't reproduce by themselves. They need a truly living

cell to commandeer for their replication. So it's not technically accurate to say that a virus lives, but only that it 'activates'. Therefore at some point in this self-assembly the virus 'activates'. It is now no longer just an inanimate microscopic lump of goo, but demonstrates many of the identifying characteristics of life itself. It is capable of reproducing and evolving, mutating to meet the challenges of its environment and surviving in the truest sense of the word. It seems impossible that an inanimate chunk of matter would all of a sudden just start combining with similar matter in the immediate neighbourhood and end up becoming active, but this is exactly the amazing process that is occurring every second of every day on the microscopic scale within and around us. It's as if a Lego set suddenly developed the ability to link itself up into a living form, and then started attacking your child.

Viruses have been defined as entities that replicate their genes inside living cells, and cause the synthesis of particles that can transfer their own genes to other cells. Viruses are composed of a nucleic acid core (consisting of either DNA or the related genetic material RNA, but not both), a protein capsid (which acts as a protective coat or shell) and occasionally an envelope membrane. That's it. No circulatory system, no lungs or gills, no digestive tract, no locomotion mechanism, and effectively not much of anything else. They can't breathe, eat, move or grow, yet they demonstrate complex and adaptive interactions with and within living cells. They can replicate, evolve and mutate within living hosts. The virus can only reproduce through a living cell, rearranging the molecules of the invaded cell into countless replicates of the viral mother. Soon the cell burgeons with newly formed viruses and ruptures, spilling thousands of viruses throughout the organism to infect many more cells and repeat the cycle.

The debate has been raging for decades as to the evolutionary history of viruses. No one knows whether viruses are chance assemblages of simpler molecules or if they were once complete, truly living parasites that over time jettisoned their cellular components to become the lean, mean killing machines they are now. Given the wide variety of viruses, both may be true. Perhaps the simpler viruses evolved from DNA or RNA and cellular proteins, while the viruses that today are more complex may have degenerated from early forms of intracellular bacteria.

One of the major facts to consider in this debate is that viruses are unable to 'survive' when not in a host, which may indicate that they must have evolved from other life forms. Or maybe not. There is a hypothesis that creatures that become parasites start losing their unneeded structures and functions. Fleas evolved from flies that dropped their wings and other unnecessary bits and pieces to spend the next few million years sucking blood. Similarly there are several functions within viruses that seem to indicate that they were once some form of bacteria that lost their cell wall and, along with it, the capacity to synthesise energy. Due to these significant and confounding factors, it is debatable whether viruses are the most complex of molecular assemblages or the simplest life forms on Earth. Did they evolve up from chunks of molecules or down from single-celled organisms? Did they just co-evolve with the rest of life? Your guess is as good as anyone else's at this point.

Virus classification is a complex system that takes into consideration the variations of structures from one virus to the other. The group names of viruses are usually in Latin or Greek and they are often named after the particular disease that only one member of that group causes. It is not a clean and simple classification system as there is ample crossover and overlap. The viruses that cause the sudden and lethal haemorrhagic fevers such as Ebola, Marburg, Dengue and others are found in three different groups: Arbovirus, Arenavirus and Filovirus. Conversely the Herpesvirus group includes not only the Herpes Simplex I virus that causes cold sores and the Herpes Simplex II that causes genital herpes, but also the Herpes Zoster that causes shingles, and the Epstein-Barr virus that causes glandular fever, as well as some cancers, and has been linked to Chronic Fatigue Syndrome ('yuppie flu').

H5N1, the particular virus that represents such an overwhelming threat to humanity, is a member of the family Orthomyxovirus. 'Ortho' means conventional and 'myxo' is mucus in Greek. However, there is nothing conventional about what this virus does to mucus membranes: attacking and literally melting them into what can only be described as bloody jelly.

The immediate threat of a global pandemic of unprecedented scale is presented by a specific form of Orthomyxovirus called influenza, Italian for 'influential visitation'. There are three different strains of the influenza virus that can infect humans, and they are named A, B and C. Most known flu cases are caused by influenza A viruses, the same family as H5N1. The influenza B and C viruses are not as widespread and primarily strike youngsters. Influenza B sometimes causes local outbreaks of flu, while influenza C rarely causes serious disease.

There are various ways viruses are transmitted between humans, primarily via inhalation or ingestion. When you are exposed to the coughs or sneezes of an infected individual the inhalation of the particles can infect you. The virus can also be transmitted by touching anything that has been in contact with the secretions of an infected person. The mechanism of infection is not through unbroken skin, but through the contact of the contaminated skin with the mouth or eyes and the subsequent ingestion. Once inside the host, the virus attacks the upper respiratory tract.

The influential visitor of particular interest is termed H5N1 after the types of surface projections on it, which make the microscopic virus look somewhat like a prickly sea urchin. There are two different types of spikes. The H stands for haemagglutinin and looks like a spear sticking up out of the surface of the virus. The N is for neuraminidase and resembles a long-stemmed mushroom. There are about 400 H spikes and 100 N mushrooms on the surface of each virus. The different types of H spikes and N mushrooms that are mixed and matched in various influenza viruses determine the name of the virus. The H5N1 virus has the fifth type of H discovered, hence H5, and the first type of N, named N1. If we were talking about the 1968 Hong Kong pandemic flu, which has the third type of H discovered with the second type of N, it would be H3N2. Nothing more complicated than that.

In fact, to keep things simple, we will continue to refer to single viruses as just that, viruses, although the proper scientific name for a single one is virion.

Microbiological nomenclatures aside, the only important factor to consider is that this particular mix of Hs and Ns is just the particular identifying characteristics of the H5N1 virus. The virus incorporates various functions and structures that give it the greatest potential to be the active agent in the coming pandemic, but one of the most significant aspects is the speed at which it evolves. It mutates at stunning speed, changing various aspects of itself in a matter of days or weeks. It is this fast-forward evolutionary capacity of H5N1 that makes it such a clear and present danger. It can mutate much faster than vaccines or pharmaceuticals can be developed, outwitting researchers at every turn. It is the ultimate moving target.

Viruses reproduce, or more accurately replicate, by commandeering the reproductive mechanism of a living cell. These structures are hidden deep within the cell's nucleus, which is a hub or centre point that serves as a command centre for the cell. In order to reach this goal the virus must somehow be able to pass its genetic material through a cell's tough and resistant membrane. Forcibly ripping through the membrane would kill the cell and spill the valuable genetic building blocks inside, so the virus has developed a very specific receptor-binding protein, a key to unlock the door to the cell without harming it. These proteins perform exactly as they are named. They bind to receptors on the living cell. They are encoded by the virus' specific genetic code and stick out from the surface like little barbs. In the influenza A viruses, they are the H spikes we discussed earlier that give H5N1 the first half of its name.

The way these receptor-binding proteins interact with the receptor is critical and usually determines what species of plant or animal the virus can infect, although some viruses, such as flu, can infect various different species. There is no universal key. There is also no universal lock, although all the locks of a particular type of tissue in a specific species are the same.

The way viruses figure out the exact combination to unlock and infect the host cell is a remarkably precise and meticulous adaptive scheme that occurs at astounding speed. A virus can mutate and evolve into a drastically different form that makes it exquisitely suitable for infecting a particular species' host within days or weeks. In evolutionary terms this is so blindingly fast that, at first glance, it doesn't really seem like random chance. The champions of intelligent design maintain that it is improbable that arbitrary attraction patterns between molecules would create a structure that responds to changes in its environment by modifying itself to a perfect fit. And it seems even more improbable that this confounding molecular assemblage would end up developing surface proteins that act as the precise key to the lock on a particular species' living cell. Thus the virus' changes may suggest 'a designer'.

Proponents of natural selection evolution, however, explain that the way a virus develops is a consequence of the vast number of mutations that arise combined with strong selection pressure, so that only those mutant viruses with the appropriate features that create a 'best fit' with their current environment will propagate and spread. They state that the virus starts with the key of the right type, albeit for a different lock, so the changes can be fairly subtle, along the lines of how a key manufacturer produces many different blanks of the same type of key to allow a wide range of combinations to be cut. Changing the H spike would be like changing the blank number. Natural selection versus intelligent design is a question that likely will not be conclusively resolved anytime soon, if ever, so you can choose your side of the debate.

An important goal for the virus is the ability to be able to infect neighbouring cells and then infect a new host.

It's this huge bottleneck that drives virus evolution, constantly developing ways to propagate and spread further and further.

Each living host cell has a specific combination that 'unlocks' it and allows the virus to inject its own genetic material into the cell nucleus. Any other combination will be unsuccessful. These lock combinations are inconceivably complex; trillions of possible configurations are possible but only one is correct. There is no bank safe on Earth that has a comparable ratio of possible wrong combinations to only one right one. Imagine that you're a bank robber and are going to try every possible combination on the bank safe to get it to open. You dial in a new one every second, 24 hours a day, 7 days a week, 365 days a year. By the end of the first year, you've dialled 31 million combinations, but the safe is still locked. To try all the possible combinations, you've only got about another 250,000 years to go. Sure, you might get lucky and hit the right combination on the first day, but you might hit a bad streak and be twirling that dial once a second for a quarter of a million years until you hit the jackpot.

Now this is assuming that you are a bank robber with intellect, perception and all the other things that go along with being a sapient creature. But this little microscopic nub of protein has beaten you from the start. It has the one right combination out of trillions for its specific host, and all of its friends have the right combination for other hosts. And it is so smart that when it meets up with some of its friends, they exchange combinations so that they can go out and open up each other's bank safes. It's like an online criminal community that breaks unbreakable bank codes and then exchanges them with each other so that they can all happily pilfer at will.

So now these dastardly viruses have the door to the bank safe open. They have full access to all the precious treasure inside. But when they get access to a living cell, exactly what are they looking for? The secret to their own reproduction.

Once the virus fits the key into the lock, the cell is fooled into 'believing' that the virus is actually something it wants, such as a hormone or nutrient. In a few minutes, the virus is accepted inside the cell walls. We all remember those horrific scenes from the movie *Alien* when the acid-spewing creatures inject their embryos into people's mouths so that they can hatch inside their guts. What the virus is doing in this case is not too unlike that particular sequence. Except that viruses are smarter than movie directors, so instead of presenting itself to the cell as a repulsive, slimy, acid-dripping *Alien* monster, it masquerades itself as something that the cell wants and needs.

In the same manner, once the virus is inside the cell, the external shell of the virus melts away and the now-exposed genetic material starts using up the matter within the living cell to make copies of itself. The virus literally disassembles the cell from the inside and uses the organic parts to make its own replicates. This process continues quickly and inexorably, soon filling up the cell with hundreds or thousands of daughter viruses.

Within six hours, the cell is completely full of H5N1 viruses and ready to burst. Once again, just as the movie alien rips out through the gut, it bursts through the wall of the mortally wounded cell, using the N mushrooms that give H5N1 the second half of its name, to release itself from the surface of the doomed cell, like a devilish baby cutting its own umbilical. Except that in the movie, there was only one offspring that blasted through the host's gut. In the real world of influenza A viruses, there are as many as thousands of newborns that issue from the doomed cell. Each one is a full-sized, fully functional exact copy of its parent. Each one is now ready to infect another living cell.

It doesn't take long for the new viruses to find another host cell and begin the six-hour process all over again. However this time there are thousands of cells being infected. And six hours later each one of these thousands of cells explode with thousands of viruses each. The number of viruses inside your body is now in the millions. And the process continues virtually exponentially in a chain reaction of replicating viruses.

Not only are there millions of viruses inside you, but also each cell that was used for the replication of viruses is now dead. The viruses are not just using up the matter of some abstract cell; they are literally eating up your body from the inside to make more copies of themselves, which will then aim to eat up even more of you.

If it stopped there at just eating you up, it would be too bad for you, but it wouldn't be too bad for general populations. The virus would nibble away at your insides until you died and that would be the end of it. But some viruses are natural-born conquerors existing to dominate new territories even more than Alexander the Great or Genghis Khan.

These viruses floating around in the bloodstream find their way out of the body in many ways. They may be coughed or sneezed out. They may come out in some bodily fluid. No matter how they exit the body, they are just lying in wait for some new, unsuspecting host to infect and start the process all over again.

The conquest of the world continues, one host at a time.

CHAPTER 3

The History of H5N1

Enveloping a world

The Great War, currently referred to as World War I, had been the greatest cataclysmic belligerence of its time. Fifteen million people lay dead, civilians and soldiers alike, as much of Europe smouldered in ruins. As peace finally dawned across a shattered continent, another source of death was on the horizon, one that would dwarf the death toll of the wars the humans had waged on each other. This was a far more ravenous reaper. It could not be shot or shelled or bombed. It was an insidious, invisible enemy who attacked in silence and stealth. It spread in the silent droplets of a sneeze and killed with the certainty of a bullet. Through its ravages, it infected almost a quarter of the population of the Earth. It killed 50 million innocent people, three times the toll of the Great War. It was known as the Spanish Flu or La Grippe. We know it as H1N1, an ancestral distant cousin of H5N1.

On a March morning in 1918, while the Great War still enveloped Europe, a company cook went to the infirmary at Camp Funston, Kansas with flu-type symptoms. By lunchtime over 100 soldiers were filling the hospital. Two days later, over 500 lay dying. Within a single week it had spread from Kansas to all 48 states and, a couple of weeks later, French civilians and military were infected, launching the disease in Europe. A few days later it reached the Orient and by May it was rampaging through South America and Africa. In the same month, over 8 million Spaniards lay dead, thus giving this disease its Hispanic nomenclature. Twenty million died in India alone.

After a brief summer respite, it returned with a vengeance in the autumn of 1918. It spread through Boston Harbour like wildfire, killing thousands. The end of the war in November and its resultant crowded victory parades created a fertile ground for dissemination of the virus. One doctor noted that people 'were dropping like flies'.

The public health systems of the world's countries were swiftly overwhelmed. Morticians had long queues and coffins were virtually impossible to find. Restrictive emergency statutes were enacted, prohibiting public gatherings, forbidding retailers from holding sales events, and even limiting funerals to a duration of a quarter of an hour. American cinemas, bars and dancehalls were shuttered. Church services were abbreviated. Some cities required certificates of health to enter and the railways refused passengers who did not have them. California's largest cities passed ordinances requiring all citizens to wear gauze masks at all times. Swiss theatres and shooting matches were closed. Britain enforced half an hour of ventilation between music hall shows. As the epidemic spread, the primary schools were closed and British streets were sprayed with disinfectants. Many ridiculous misconceptions of the time were championed as fact. Porridge sales soared as it was believed that it contained some mysterious anti-flu element. Some industries and offices changed their no-smoking rules and encouraged workers to smoke. Why? They were under the mistaken impression that tobacco smoke could kill the flu virus.

Influenza typically attacks the very young and old. The reason is that over time humans develop a significant number of special proteins called antibodies to several different influenza strains, each antibody correlating to a previous infection. Antibodies bind themselves to specific viral proteins. When an influenza virus enters the human body, the antibodies bind the H spike, blocking this 'key' so that it won't fit the living cell's 'lock'. Another group of antibodies bind to the N mushroom to prevent the release of newly formed viruses from the first commandeered host cell. Each antibody we have protects us from reinfection with that particular strain of influenza, but is unable to bind to new strains. In these cases, new antibodies must be developed, hopefully in time before the virus ravages and kills the person.

As we age, however, our immune system has a tendency to weaken. It has increasing difficulty in fighting off new strains and no longer has such a good 'memory' about what influenzas it has fought off before. So it is possible for the same strain to reinfect an old person. This is in marked contrast to younger, healthier people, who cannot be reinfected by the same strain as their antibodies still have excellent 'memory'. In the case of very young people, their immune system may be strong and vigorous but they have not yet fought off many strains so their immune system's 'memory' doesn't have much in it to remember.

One of the factors that made the Spanish Flu so fearsome was that it atypically did not follow the conventional pattern of influenza A in primarily attacking the young and old. For reasons that have never been adequately explained, many of the victims were in their 20s.

The first symptoms of a patient with Spanish flu were the usual ones we now correlate with what we know as the flu: high fever, sore throat, dry cough, headache and body pains. These symptoms appeared quite viciously in some individuals, who were struck down with severe symptoms within minutes. In less than a week pneumonia would surface, driving fever upwards and forcing the continuous issuance of bloody sputum. Death via a series of complications usually came swiftly.

Anecdotes abound of New York subway passengers entering the train healthy and dying in convulsions, spewing foamy blood, before the end of the line. Four women played bridge well into the night. Three of them died by morning. Ocean liners crossing the Atlantic arrived with one out of every dozen passengers dead. Victims were dying in the street, in stores, in offices, in military barracks, turning blue and struggling for air as they suffocated in bloody froth.

The global effects of this pandemic were unprecedented and exceeded even that of the Black Death of the mid 14th century. It single-handedly lowered the average lifespan in the US and Europe by ten years. The Spanish Flu may even have changed the course of international history. Pacifist US President Woodrow Wilson had been disabled by flu during the negotiations for the Treaty of Versailles that ended World War I. Had he been able to participate, the treaty would certainly have been more humanitarian and equitable. However, in his absence, the final form of the treaty drafted by the triumphant Allies was so punitive and restrictive for the defeated side that a decade later an unemployed Austrian painter sought to strike back against the Allies who had imposed these excesses on his people. Thus Adolf Hitler began the march to World War II.

The pandemic followed its human carriers to every corner of the earth. The return of military personnel to their home countries gave this virus a free ride to new horizons to ravage. At first it was believed that this disease was a biological weapon the Germans had unleashed upon Allied troops. Soon it was recognised that it was an airborne infectious agent and medical researchers around the world mobilised to come up with some way of destroying this vicious nemesis.

Many of the treatments were ineffective and seem ridiculous in the eyes of modern science. Carbolic acid mixed with quinine or sodium bicarbonate with boric acid was sprayed in noses. This did nothing to the infection but certainly caused significant discomfort to the poor patient. However, the new 'germ theory' pioneered by Koch and Pasteur was beginning to take root and the standards that we now take for granted were being introduced by luminaries such as Lister: sequestration of infected individuals; periodic disinfection of hospital areas, utensils and cups; and frequent handwashing with antiseptic solutions.

O'Malley and Hartman were the first to discuss injecting infected patients with the serum from others who were convalescent: the first real-world application of antibodies boosting the immune system that had just been described by Erhlich. Until this time, there was no clear delineation between viruses and bacteria and the terms were used interchangeably. Nicolle and Le Bailly first suggested that the infection was caused by viruses that could pass through a filter that captured bacteria, thus they had to be significantly smaller. Their test results proved Koch was correct and they were able to duplicate human disease in animals. However, they still did not comprehend that viruses used the human cell for their own reproduction, a key discovery that along with greater understanding of the immune system led to the widespread use of vaccines, as traditional antibiotics are useless against viruses.

There are now several major types of viral vaccines, but they all work in essentially the same way. Partial, weakened or killed virus is injected into the human body. This usually triggers a mild infection. The immune system seeks out the vaccine elements and destroys them while adding their description to the body's 'memory bank' of known agents. When a virulent and dangerous example of the same virus invades the body, the immune system can respond quickly and accurately by inactivating the virus before it can infect cells or once a cell is infected by destroying that cell.

Many years after the tide of Spanish Flu ebbed, human virus samples that had been saved from the pandemic demonstrated that it was much more closely related to avian viruses than anyone expected, raising the possibility that it arose directly by mutation into a type that can infect humans. The analyses of the Spanish Flu virus show that H5N1 shares many of the types of mutations that its 1918 counterpart had, compared to traditional avian viruses. It is suspected that these very mutations allowed the development of the incredibly virulent agent that killed 50 million people.

Variations of bird flu struck in 1957 (H2N2) and 1968 (H3N2). These were much milder, but still killed approximately 2 million people each. In each of these cases, a virus that originated in birds mixed genes with a human flu and the epidemic began.

By 1959, early versions of H5N1 struck Scotland's bird population. This wave soon petered out and didn't surface again until 32 years later in turkeys south of the border in England. However, the first recorded transmission of H5N1 from birds to humans occurred in Hong Kong in 1997, infecting 18 people and killing 6 of them. Prompt action from the local authorities included slaughtering every chicken in the territory within three days and the virus was stopped.

A major outbreak of H5N1 hit Thailand and Vietnam's poultry population in January 2004 and within weeks was present in several neighbouring Asian countries, including China, Indonesia and Japan. More than 40 million chickens were destroyed and the spread was contained two months later, after 23 people had died. In the midst of this outbreak the virus was detected in Vietnamese pigs, echoing events that are believed to precede pandemics. In July 2004 H5N1 surfaced in Thailand and China again, and the next month spread to Malaysia. Many more chickens were destroyed to stem this tide. By January 2005, half of the Vietnamese cities and provinces were infected and millions more poultry were sacrificed. In all almost 200 million birds have died or been slaughtered, yet H5N1 marches inexorably onwards.

H5N1 is now present in hundreds of millions of Asian food birds that transmit it through faeces on their feathers, eggs and cages. Since the virus is airborne, infection is inevitable. Some birds show no symptoms, while being highly contagious, making the disease difficult to spot. The virus can survive for a month in refrigerated poultry and indefinitely if frozen.

In the spring 2005 cases in Thailand and Vietnam, the first human-to-human spread was discovered (although it was still being debated if it was bird-to-human). However, what worries researchers most is that the mortality rate of the disease in these cases has dropped by half to about one third of those infected, down from three-quarters. While this may seem to be good news, it is indeed quite the opposite; a drop in the human mortality rate has indicated in the past that the virus is evolving closer to the stage where it can launch a global pandemic. There are reasons found in the very structure of the virus that dictate that, as it becomes better adapted to human-to-human transmission, its lethality rate falls, but in total it kills far more people as it spreads to thousands or millions of times more humans. The Spanish Flu killed 50 million people, while infecting a billion. Various researchers have agreed that experiments indicate H5N1 is increasing its human-infectiousness qualities very quickly and that a pandemic could be just around the corner. One of the leading researchers, Dr Robert Webster of St Jude Children's Research Hospital, has stated: 'This is the worst virus I have ever met in my entire career.' Dr Anthony Fauci, director of the US National Institute of Allergy and Infectious Diseases has said, 'This virus has the potential to trigger the next pandemic, which, judging from history, is well overdue.'

By the late summer of 2005 H5N1 had spread right across Asia, leaving a large swath of dead birds across southern Russia. Then the news arrived that the birds had entered Europe.

At the same time, due to erratic enforcement, Vietnam's poultry control measures had not slowed the rate of infection. Poultry was banned from all cities from last year but in Ho Chi Minh City (formerly Saigon) chickens are still a common sight in the streets. A recent study discovered that more than 70 per cent of ducks and geese in the

Mekong Delta tested positive for influenza, thus the Vietnamese government ordered the slaughter of 1.5 million of them. Farmers had been offered only a fraction of the birds' value in compensation so almost all those birds are still alive at the time of writing. In Indonesia, researchers found that half of all the pigs in some regions were infected with H5N1. Since pigs are a common 'mixing vessel' for bird viruses to hybridise into versions that can be spread via human-to-human contact, this ominous news also led to significant concern that H5N1 could make the final adaptation to a truly human virus somewhere in Indonesia.

The evidence grew day by day that the virus might have begun to change into one capable of ready transmission between humans and of causing a full-blown pandemic. Andrew D Pavia, MD, chairman of the Infectious Disease Society Task Force on Influenza, stated:

> We believe that the next influenza pandemic is imminent. These predictions are primarily based upon the historic intervals between outbreaks as well as the increased spread and ominous behaviour of the H5N1 avian influenza virus, which now is endemic among birds in much of Asia. We are very concerned that the H5N1 avian virus has shown the ability to mutate and has become capable of infecting mammals, including pigs, tigers, cats, and humans as well as birds.

Within days the World Health Organization (WHO) had issued a report:

> It is possible that the avian H5N1 viruses are becoming more infectious for people, facilitating infection in a

greater number or range of people. The changes are all consistent with the avian virus possibly adapting to a human host.

This backed up WHO's earlier statement:

> The simultaneous occurrence in several countries of large epidemics of highly pathogenic H5N1 influenza in domestic poultry is historically unprecedented. The present situation may grow worse. The potential for further spread of ongoing poultry epidemics, both within affected countries and to other countries, is therefore great. Of all the avian influenza viruses, which normally cause infection in birds and pigs only, the H5N1 strain may have a unique capacity to cause severe disease, with high mortality, in humans.

US Centers for Disease Control and Prevention (CDC) researchers recreated a complete Spanish Flu virus by gathering viral DNA from the preserved tissues of victims, including an Alaskan woman who was frozen in 1918. The analysis shows that the Spanish Flu is an avian influenza virus that evolved into a human one, an evolutionary process eerily similar to H5N1. Jeffery K Taubenberger, chief of molecular pathology at the US Armed Forces Institute of Pathology and one of the CDC study leaders stated 'the fact that [gene] changes identified in the 1918 analysis are also seen in H5N1 . . . suggests that these changes may facilitate virus replication in human cells and increase pathogenicity.'

The clock is ticking. We may be minutes from midnight and not even know it.

CHAPTER 4

How Can This Pandemic Start?

A shroud of dirty feathers

Influenza viruses have developed an insidious ability to mutate at staggering speed. H5N1 now has the ability to cross species' barriers from birds, infecting cats, horses and pigs. But that is not the worst of it. All that it is waiting for is to infect some particular unsuspecting human who is already infected with some form of human influenza. Then H5N1 will use the common ability of influenza viruses to 'swap' particular parts of itself with the human influenza virus infecting the human host. The resultant evolved H5N1 will then be as contagious among humans as a common cold or regular flu. It will be able to be spread widely and easily by coughing, sneezing or touch.

Influenza A viruses can 'swap' or 'reorganise' genetic materials from each other and merge into a completely new and previously unknown virus. This reorganisation process is known as 'antigenic shift' as the genes shift from one virus to another. The resultant new virus has the ability to infect species that it previously could not, as the immune systems of populations have no existing antibodies to fight off an agent that they have never encountered before.

How Can This Pandemic Start?

Historically this antigenic shifting has resulted in global pandemics with very high mortalities. In order for this to occur, the bird form of the H5N1 has to appropriate genes from another type of influenza A virus. Sometimes the antigenic shift occurs in pigs, with bird flu strains latching onto a pig flu virus that can very easily be passed to humans; thus it has everything it needs to make the leap to a fully human disease. But H5N1 can also take the more direct route and use people as the 'mixing vessel' to re-engineer itself into the most supremely efficient killer of our times.

Let's consider the case of a hypothetical Chinese poultry farmer who was afflicted years ago with an influenza such as H3N2. This virus was responsible for the Hong Kong flu epidemic in the late 1960s but still widely circulates today. Our farmer suffered no long-lasting ill effects and the 'dormant' H3N2 has been lurking somewhere in his body ever since. He is constantly in the presence of his chickens and ducks, exposed on a daily basis to their faeces, which contain billions of H5N1 viruses in an easily spread airborne form. If you were to visit some Third World family poultry farms you would be astounded at the lack of hygienic conditions. People literally live with their poultry, and in many cases the birds freely roam in and out of the farmhouse. Faeces, feathers and bird bits are everywhere, on every surface, on shoes. I even saw bird droppings on dinner plates. Infected birds can excrete virus for almost two weeks so it's only a matter of time until our farmer is infected with the H5N1 bird virus.

Once the H5N1 bird virus is in his body, it will meet up with the H3N2 human virus and, in the nefarious manner these viruses have evolved, they will 'shift' some genes

from one to the other. The H5N1 bird virus will appropriate from the H3N2 human virus the exact combination for
the human cell 'lock' that the human virus has used in the
past to infect our farmer. He has now become a 'mixing
vessel' in which genetic information from human virus to
bird virus has been exchanged. The resultant H5N1 still
has the same horrific symptoms of melting the body from
the inside and a fearsome mortality rate. But now it also
has the key to the farmer's cells. It has become a human-
to-human-spreadable lethal disease on the launch pad to a
pandemic.

When the H5N1 mixes with, say, an H3N2, the result
may not be an H5N1 at all. It might emerge as an H5N2 or
an H3N1 (taking the H from one and the N from the
other). Therefore the actual name of the virus that causes
the pandemic may not be H5N1 at all. But it will definitely
originate from the H5N1 bird virus, thus we're sticking to
that name throughout this book.

Now the H5N1 has the combination to the human cell,
it will attack it, force it to make endless copies of itself and
our farmer will become contagious. He will likely show
no symptoms for at least a day, and all the while he is
shedding millions of newly 'humanised' H5N1 viruses
everywhere he goes. During that time his family, friends,
neighbours, even the people at the feed store will have no
clue that he is making them the earliest links in the pandemic to come. He hasn't even sniffled or sneezed once.
Yet every time he shakes hands, every time he shares a cup
of water, everything he touches passes the 'new and
improved' H5N1 along.

By the time the next morning dawns and he is feeling
feverish and achy with a scratchy throat, dry cough and
the usual flu symptoms, he has already possibly infected

most of the people he has seen in the previous day. And they are infecting the people they meet. And the people they meet.

One of them travels to Beijing, a metropolitan area housing more than 13 million people, to sell his chickens. He casually passes the H5N1 along to the other people in the poultry market, the other sellers and his customers. These people go on to have lunch at a crowded restaurant, go to see a movie in a packed cinema, or just stroll along Beijing's swarming streets. At every encounter, each person increases the spread of the virus onto others. One of the market customers sits on a bus next to a businessperson scheduled to fly to London the next morning. At Beijing Airport flights are leaving for destinations all over the world. More than 300 flights will leave on this day, and our businessperson comes into contact with several passengers who will shortly be on some of these flights. Then he sits in a 747 with 400 other people for 11 hours. He uses the toilet a couple of times, chats with the person sitting next to him. The flight attendants take away his used dishes and cups. Then he arrives at London Heathrow Airport, where he comes into contact with many other people, some of whom will be travelling on a number of Heathrow's 1,300 daily flights. It's all over.

It's been about a week since our poultry farmer began shedding the virus and the epidemic has become a pandemic. His unique H5N1 strain is now in dozens of countries and spreading fast. If the Spanish Flu could permeate all 48 US states in a single week in 1918 when the fastest way to travel from coast to coast was a train, just imagine the velocity of the spread of H5N1 in the jet age.

Even if our original farmer, who by this time is showing severe symptoms of H5N1 infection, is immediately quarantined, the damage has been done. H5N1 has escaped from Pandora's Box. Our farmer has served as the 'mixing vessel', the missing link that H5N1 was waiting for to become a fully human disease pandemic.

Influenza A typically infects the upper respiratory tract, basically the throat and upper lungs. The reason for this is due to the fact that these tissues have receptors for the influenza virus built right into them. These receptors perform other important physiological functions for the host. However, viruses have taken advantage of the presence of these structures by evolving the ability to use critical molecules as receptors. The host can't simply eliminate or mutate these receptors into other forms without losing their critical function, thus the virus has an effective point of entry.

There are countless ways to be infected with an influenza A virus. Touch something, anything at all, that has been in contact with an infected individual. Then rub the moist corners of your eyes, nose or mouth – an involuntary reaction each of us does dozens of times a day. You're infected. It is not obligatory to inhale the airborne particles from an infected person sneezing or coughing on you. Think of that next time you use a public toilet, pick up something from the pavement, or are even handed coins as change. Let's not even mention visiting bars and restaurants.

On a recent trip to Rome, I observed the barista at a trendy Via Veneto coffee house 'washing' the cups. His process was to take the dirty cups, drop them into a sink of standing, slimy, soapy water just enough to rinse out whatever coffee was left in them, and then put them on a drip tray to dry. I ordered several espressos just to carefully examine the cups, certainly not to put them anywhere near my lips. As I thought, I found lipstick on most of them, several different colours on some. Now if the lipstick is still there, what makes you think that the viruses carried by that individual coffee-lover would not be? Soapy water standing until it is lukewarm is not bleach. It does not disinfect anything on contact.

So the next time your cup or glass or fork seems a bit spotted or soiled, ask yourself what are the chances that a virus is not hitching a ride on it? Remember that it would take a thousand viruses to stretch across the diameter of one of your hairs. Imagine just how many can be lurking on that little spot on your cup.

At the Via Veneto coffee bar, I also observed how many cups the barista had and how many coffees he was serving. I calculated that he reused each cup, on average, once every 20 minutes. Given that these bars are open 18 hours a day, if only one H5N1 infected person has a cup of espresso with his sunrise breakfast, his unsterilised cup will be used by 53 other people just in that one day.

An interesting development has historically occurred with influenza A viruses. As they become more and more adept at human-to-human transmission, their mortality rates drop dramatically. That is quite likely an evolutionary adaptation to allow the host species to continue. At first it seems absurd that the drop in the mortality rate should indicate the beginning of a pandemic. It would seem to be logical that the higher the mortality rate, the more devastating the pandemic. Influenza A viruses defy logic and this is just one more case.

If a virus such as H5N1 that in the past killed three out of every four people it infects were to become easily spread from person to person, it could create a situation where the very species it preys upon would be exterminated. All it would take is a few pandemics back-to-back at a 75 per cent mortality rate and *Homo sapiens* would likely soon go the way of the dinosaurs. It seems as if there is a delicate balancing act between the virus' requirement to attack living cells to replicate and the number of individuals in a particular species that it kills. It may be that once it has the combination to the particular 'lock', it is just trying to preserve its own survival by ensuring that there will always be populations of this species to infect. After all, no virus can continue to survive without a host species.

The first outbreaks of H5N1 had a human mortality rate of 73 per cent and most recently they are down to approximately 35 per cent. This ratio is watched very carefully, as when the mortality rate drops below 10 per cent it is generally agreed that the conditions are ripe for pandemic spread.

Efficiency of transmission is the key factor in a pandemic. The easier it is for one person to spread the virus to another person, then the faster the pandemic will spread. When H5N1 killed 73 per cent of all the people it infected, it was primarily a bird-only virus. It was quite difficult for humans to be infected. They literally had to be in constant contact with bird faeces and sooner or later, begrudgingly, the bird virus would concede to infect and kill them, since the human immune systems had no hope of recognising what these new strange viruses were.

Along the way, the bird virus started to recombine and pick up mammalian characteristics. A characteristic here, a characteristic there. Thus the bird virus started to become a bit more recognisable to the human immune system and the mortality rate began to drop until it is now down to 35 per cent. We have seen that H5N1 needs to 'swap' genes with a truly human influenza virus in order to become a pandemic. Naturally, it depends what genes it swaps. In one particular individual it might swap genes that make it incredibly easy to transmit from person to person, yet only cause a bit of fever and a sniffle or two. In which case, the gene 'swapping' has created a disease that is less virulent, or vicious, than the parents. This is not unlike two fit, tall human parents who have a short, obese offspring. It can happen.

However, in many viral cases, the offspring takes on the best characteristics of the parents. H5N1 would tend to take on as many of the 'easy spread' genes of the human influenza virus, while abandoning as few of its own 'massive mortality' genes in the process. We know from previous pandemics that the optimum balance of these factors is reached when the human mortality rate reaches just below 10 per cent. That seems to be the perfect viral gene mix of the profile of a pandemic. Enough genes present to kill just under 10 per cent of the infected population virtually ensures that the rest of the genes for immediate and widespread transmission are there as well. Instead of 73 per cent or 35 per cent of a few dozen people, we have just under 10 per cent of a few billion. That is the profile of the pandemic that may ravage the world.

CHAPTER 5

What You Can Do Now to Help Keep Yourself Safe

First of all: Don t panic!

Use this as your new mantra: Don't panic. Don't panic. Don't panic. I know that reading this book may convince you that we're all going to die tomorrow. If you panic, however, you will not be taking the proper precautions and you may be in even greater danger than if you had done nothing at all.

This book contains literally hundreds of precautions that *can* be taken. However, I doubt whether the most germophobic reader is going to implement each and every one of them. You are not 'The Boy in the Bubble'. It is simply inconsistent with any measure of 'normal' social human life to become obsessed with sealing every imaginable vector of germs into your system. It's not possible, not feasible, and not even desirable.

Remember: Moderation in all things, including moderation. Be aware of what is happening, keep your eyes and ears open, become a news junkie, be prepared, have courage and react to situations as they occur. Keep a cool head and keep your pandemic preparations on standby. Implement some of the precautions in this book that you can reasonably fit into your current lifestyle, but don't go overboard. Sure, you can catch the next plane to the Canadian tundra and live off Saskatoon berries and charred moose meat, but that would be a big waste of time if the pandemic fizzles out before it starts.

The majority of the suggestions in this book are at least somewhat related to common sense. A small number of them are wacko off-the-wall precautions that only the most extreme, paranoid germophobic nutcase would even remotely consider. I have a responsibility to present all of these to you and let you choose which, if any, you will adopt.

The pandemic could happen. It could ravage the Earth within weeks in ways that are even worse than we can imagine. Or it may simply never materialise. A rather likely possibility is that it could flare up in some far-off corner of the world and be stopped in its tracks by prompt action by local medical authorities. International mobilisation is being prepared to be able to rush massive amounts of antiviral and vaccine (once it is available) to swamp any geographical area where there is an H5N1 flare-up. Maybe that will snuff out the pandemic before it can begin. Maybe it won't. The bottom line is that we don't know until it happens. It certainly is not going to hurt you to be prepared within reason.

Keep in mind that these worst possible case scenarios have a very tiny percentage possibility of ever occurring. This pandemic may never come. Don't worry yourself into an early grave over the prospect.

You can implement any of these precautions at any time up to the time the pandemic strikes. Some of the simpler ones are basic hygienic and infection-prevention common sense, and you would be well advised to start following as many of them as possible right now. However, I don't expect anyone to start spending thousands on complex home electronic air disinfection equipment until there is a clear and present danger.

Avoid infection on crowded buses, in schools, offices and other public areas

What do Donald Trump, Prince Charles and Saddam Hussein have in common? They don't like shaking hands with you. Saddam was reputed to have had visitors disinfect their hands and clothing before they met him. Donald and the prince simply shun any direct physical contact to avoid germs and will go to some lengths to keep from being touched. Among famous historical germophobes we can include billionaire Howard Hughes, physics genius Nikola Tesla and Adolf Hitler.

I hate to agree with Hitler or Saddam on anything but, when it comes to taking precautions in the H5N1 age, I'm afraid that I have to concur.

There are many times when it cannot be helped but to come into contact with a large number of potentially infectious people. In an H5N1 pandemic situation, each and every person must be considered as a possible source of infection. Remember that an individual does not necessarily have to demonstrate any outward symptoms to be transmitting H5N1. So it's just simply not good enough to shy from people who are sneezing, sniffling and blowing their nose. The person next to you could be fully H5N1 contagious although they look and act perfectly healthy.

You would actually be surprised how many people you come into contagious proximity with every day. Here are some examples:

Homemaker on shopping day: 100
Commuter on train, day in office: 400
Commuter on train, day running errands in city: 1,200
Sports fan in stadium: 1,500
City bus driver: 1,800
Airline counter staff at airport: 3,500
Ticket seller at underground train station: 5,000
Refreshment seller in stadium: 8,500
Outdoor newspaper seller in city: 10,000
Exhibitor at major trade show: 15,000
Club-crawler in Ibiza: 20,000
Tourist visiting Las Vegas casinos: 32,000

Now let's do a little maths. Let's assume that each of these people is out doing their thing ten hours a day. And let's also assume that we are in the midst of a full-blown pandemic. Here is a rudimentary approximation of the odds on coming home at the end of that day without getting infected:

Homemaker on shopping day: 1 to 1
Commuter on train, day in office: 4 to 1
Commuter on train, day running errands in city: 12 to 1
Sports fan in stadium: 15 to 1
City bus driver: 18 to 1
Airline counter staff at airport: 35 to 1
Ticket seller at underground train station: 50 to 1
Refreshment seller in stadium: 85 to 1
Outdoor newspaper seller in city: 100 to 1
Exhibitor at major trade show: 150 to 1
Club-crawler in Ibiza: 200 to 1
Tourist visiting Las Vegas casinos: 320 to 1

Now especially for the Las Vegas visitor, I'm sure that they would never place a bet of a single dollar where their chances of winning were 1 and their chances of losing were 319!

You must consider any surface or location that is frequented by masses of people to be highly infectious. Anywhere you go in your daily life, including transport, work, stores, restaurants and leisure facilities, you can be assured that many other people have already visited. And wherever people have been, they have left their H5N1 behind.

Much of this relates to how hard the pandemic hits. It is clear in the later chapters on government-planned response that, should the pandemic be as pervasive as feared, it would follow that there would be bans on gatherings considered not strictly vital, including sport, recreation, schooling, trade shows and conventions. It is possible that non-essential work be brought to a halt and travel be severely restricted even within the country itself. There is no doubt that under such a fearsome weight of pandemic and the accompanying panic, life will change radically.

No one can know the future and with all the well-intentioned planning in the world, the devil is always in the details. Much of this advice may be rendered irrelevant by government-imposed pandemic policies. However, not all countries in the world will act in unison of policy or timing. For every stable, efficient developed country with a well thought-out and implementable pandemic policy there is a country such as Somalia, which has not had the merest form of government for years. By all means adhere to your own government's pandemic policy but, if you find it falls short of optimal, here are some tips that may help you stay safe.

What You Can Do Now

Transport

- Try to adopt flexible hours so that your commute is not at peak travel times, minimising the number of people you will be forced into close proximity with.
- If someone sits next to you on a bus or train, stand and move to a less crowded area.
- Never sit facing anyone. Sit so you are facing the same direction as the person in front of you.
- Don't stand in the crowd trying to get on the bus or train first. Let them all go in and then get on at the last minute.
- Take the window seat rather than the aisle. That will keep you away from the crowded aisle.
- Keep the window open if you can to breathe in fresh, uncontaminated air. If that is not possible then leave your seat and stand by the door, especially if its window can be opened.
- Shun public transport if you can and travel in your own vehicle.

Work

- If people at work are becoming ill with H5N1, call in sick even though you may not be, even at the cost of getting fired.
- Telecommute if you can.
- Avoid meetings and conferences. Shun trade shows and conventions at all costs.
- Sit as far away from your fellow workers as feasible. Keep the maximum distance possible away from visiting salesmen, engineers, consultants, etc.

- If you work facing someone else, see if you can turn your desk or workstation around to face away from them.
- Keep as many people out of your cubicle or office as possible.
- Don't ever use anyone else's cup, glass or utensils.
- Cover your hand with a paper towel when using the fax, photocopier or other much-used office equipment.
- Don't share your tools, utensils, or own equipment with anyone else. Don't let anyone use your computer, desk or work area.
- If you have your own office, work with the door closed and the window open if you can, even in winter.
- Don't attend the office party or go out for a drink after work.
- Avoid the lunchroom or canteen. Eat at your desk.
- If you work in retail, direct sales or any other job that causes you to meet a lot of different people, ask for a transfer to a desk job.
- Be especially careful if you work in the poultry or swine industry.

Schools

- Pick a seat at the back of the class as far from other students as possible.
- Go to the most secluded part of the library to study.
- Stay away from groups of people during class changes or breaks.
- Avoid working in groups.

- Pack your lunch and eat it alone.
- For sports lessons, bring your own towel and keep it in your bag until you need it. Always wear sandals or flip-flops in the shower and changing room. Bring your own soap and shampoo.
- Clean lab equipment prior to use, or hold a tissue when you touch it.
- If H5N1 is in your school, consider online or correspondence courses.

Risk assessment is a difficult task for the average worker or scholar. It is effectively inevitable that you will come into contact with a large number of people in the work or school setting. The best thing that anyone can do is to keep a close eye on the progress of H5N1 through the news media in order to gauge when and how to implement some of these suggestions. Your employer or school administration should be polled for their policy on issuing respirators and other infection control gear, increasing the airflow in closed-in areas, implementing higher levels of hygiene in the buildings, allowing telecommuting, or even restructuring the places where people congregate. You may even want to volunteer at your school or workplace to educate your fellows on basic hygiene and infection control procedures.

We're not talking about catching a cold here. H5N1 isn't your typical garden variety little bug that gives you the sniffles for a couple of days and then goes away. H5N1 is lethal. Some estimates state that it could kill over 5 per cent of the entire population of the world. That's more than four times the number of people killed in World Wars I and II combined. One person out of twenty could be in a grave within months. You don't want to be one of them. This is not the time to ignore or ridicule efforts to keep yourself safe. You are not a germophobic Jerry Seinfeld clone if you practise reasonable safety precautions. If people want to laugh at you for being paranoid, let them. You may be laughing last!

The most germ-laden public environment of them all

There are ways to stay safe from infection without moving to a desert island. They are simple, straightforward, common-sense tips that can save you from contracting a horrible and potentially deadly illness. Let's start at the most critical contamination point: the public lavatory.

Studies have shown that viruses can indeed exist on public bathroom surfaces for an hour or longer. The toilet seat is far from the only source of contamination. H5N1 can be found on surfaces within the cubicle, on the toilet paper (especially if it's wet, which makes it a better environment for the virus) and on the floor. There are virtually no bathroom surfaces where H5N1 can't be transmitted. This virus can be present on doorknobs, flush handles and taps, and can infect you whenever you touch your now-contaminated hands to your eyes, nose or mouth.

Germs can also be shot into the air when a toilet flushes. The resulting spray can douse the toilet seat and even the sink, doors and wall with a shower of microscopic germ-laden droplets. Studies have shown that the spray from a flushing toilet with the lid up can spray out over 3.7 metres.

Experts agree that one of the best ways to protect yourself in a public bathroom or from viruses no matter where you are is to wash your hands very thoroughly. Hand-washing works because the friction of rubbing your hands together in the presence of a water 'wettening' compound such as soap loosens germs from your skin and traps them in the foamy lather. When you rinse away the lather, you're rinsing away the germs.

There are precautions to take when facing the pervasive contamination in a public bathroom:

- Avoid using toilets that haven't been flushed. Don't use a toilet seat that looks dirty or wet. Urine usually contains only harmless bacteria when it leaves the body but it can shield live virus.
- If they're available, use paper seat covers. If not, then cover the seat with toilet paper. There's no point putting paper or tissue down on a wet seat as the germs will just be transmitted right to your skin. Dry the seat first, even if you have to use up half a roll of toilet paper to keep any liquid from ever touching your hands.
- There is always the option to not sit down on a toilet seat. Both men and women in good physical condition can adopt a position that looks like they're caught halfway from standing up from a chair and hold that long enough to complete their business. The anatomical construction of males is somewhat more fortunate than that of females as they can urinate standing up. However, there are new products that enable women to do the same. They are disposable funnel-type devices and, if you can get past the comical aspects, they are excellent ways to enable females to urinate while standing up and facing the toilet.
- Don't ever place your purse, briefcase, bags or packages on the floor or on top of the toilet tank. Use the hook, if one is available, or hold them in your hands.

- Wet hands and lather well with soap. Work the lather evenly from one hand to the other. Hot or warm water is preferable to cold, not because it kills bacteria and viruses (water hot enough to do that would scald you) but because the soap lathers better with it. You should spend at least 15 seconds rubbing your hands together after they're wet and lathered (about the amount of times it takes to sing the 'Happy Birthday' song twice) and even more if your hands are especially dirty. Then rinse your hands with a stream of clear running water until all the lather is washed away.

- After washing, dry your hands thoroughly with paper towels when available. Paper towels allow you to properly dry your hands and if there is decent waste disposal available they pose negligible risk to your health. When you use a rolling cloth towel fixture assure yourself that the part of the towel you dry your hands on has not been used before. When these towels get stuck or reach the end of the roll, it's easy to end up using the same portion someone else has used already. Try to avoid using hot-air dryers. Most of them are unsanitary because they pull their air not from the outside but from the bathroom floor, which even in a clean facility is teeming with germs. Also avoid using a common towel, which has been contaminated by an unknown number of hands. Dry hands with an emergency supply of tissues or use toilet paper.

- Don't touch your eyes, nose or mouth until you have washed and dried your hands thoroughly. Don't touch anything directly. People come to the sink with contaminated hands, turn on the water and, after they wash, touch the dirty faucet handle again. Turn off the taps and open the door only with a paper towel or tissue. Remember that only 15 per cent of all people wash their hands after using a public toilet!

Sanitise your hands and face without water, anywhere and anytime

Both US President George W Bush and Vice President Dick Cheney immediately apply alcohol hand sanitiser as soon as they can after shaking hands or coming into contact with anyone. In their positions, they have to be in contact with a large number of people, often from every country in the world, thus they are taking reasonable precautions.

Alcohol hand-rub, gel or rinse sanitisers are portable, effective disinfectants containing at least 60 per cent alcohol with emollients to keep your skin from drying or chapping. Washing hands with warm water and soap is still the most effective method to reduce the number of germs on your hands. However, alcohol hand sanitisers are indicated after washing hands with soap and water as an additional step to kill germs or when soap and water handwashing is not feasible.

These products are marketed in small, convenient, containers with built-in dispensers. To use the product, put an amount the size of a small coin in the palm of your hand and carefully rub your hands all over, including underneath the fingernails.

Alcohol-based products are not as effective on visible soil so, if your hands are clearly dirty, wash your hands using warm water and soap and dry them completely before applying the alcohol hand products. The alcohol in the compound will completely evaporate in about 10 to 15 seconds, leaving your hands clean and dry. Immediately after the alcohol hand sanitiser product has dried on your skin, it is perfectly safe to handle food products, touch your eyes, nose, mouth, etc.

There are various reasons why alcohol hand sanitisers are becoming so popular:

- They reduce the number of bacteria better than washing with soap and water and are more effective than washing with an antibacterial soap, even the hospital formulations (unless your hands are particularly dirty).
- They are less time-consuming and more convenient, which can lead people to clean their hands more often than they would with soap and water.
- They will not assist microbes obtaining resistance to the product because there is no alcohol residue, so it isn't around long enough for a significant amount of the germs to mutate.

The various alcohol hand sanitisers on the market differ significantly from one another. The products that are composed of a thick gel or foam are preferred as they will prevent dripping and will maximise the critical contact of alcohol to the surface of the skin during cleaning. The effectiveness of the sanitiser is also related to the type and amount of alcohol incorporated in the formulation. A range of 60 to 70 per cent alcohol is considered the most effective percentage to minimise contamination on the hands. Ethanol is generally considered superior in its virucidal effects to isopropanol, however both types of alcohol are sufficiently effective in inactivating and eliminating germs.

Unfortunately, alcohol is flammable at the concentrations found in hand sanitisers and reports of fire accidents are already surfacing. All alcohol hand sanitisers are classified as hazardous materials; those formulated primarily with ethanol being more flammable than those containing isopropanol or mixtures of ethanol and isopropanol. However, as long as they are used sensibly and are stored away from high temperatures, sparks or flames, their benefits far outweigh any risks from flammability. Alcohol hand sanitisers are readily available and very affordable.

Sterilise the part of your hand that contains thousands of germs

You've washed your hands according to all the advice and even used an alcohol hand sanitiser as a 'chaser'. Now you look at your squeaky clean hands and don't realise that you may have thousands of germs still on them – underneath your fingernails.

The dirt under your fingernails can harbour countless germs even when your hands are spotlessly clean. The area under the fingernails is a reservoir for micro-organisms. Unless cleaning under the nails occurs daily with a nail file, nail brush or even an old bristly toothbrush you can quickly get a build-up of dead skin cells, soil and other assorted dirt that acts as a cosy home for literally thousands of bacteria and viruses. Germs love dark, moist areas with lots of filth around and under your fingernails is a perfect breeding ground for them.

A healthy fingernail is one that is clean, short, with any jagged nail tips filed down to smoothness and with the surrounding cuticle and skin fully intact. Long manicured fingernails may look pretty on the ladies, but when it comes to controlling infection in a pandemic period, a fingernail that extends beyond the fingertip is just too long.

Women with artificial nails, nail extensions, nail jewellery and piercing are giving bacteria a wonderful place to reproduce. And they will reproduce very quickly, leading to bacterial counts in the hundreds or thousands. Viruses won't reproduce under your nails but they will hide out there for far longer than you might think, active and waiting to infect you when you scratch, have broken skin or touch your eyes, nose or mouth. Germs are not just living under your fingernails, but under the nails of the people around you as well. When you meet someone with long fingernails, consider them to be contagious and don't shake their hands or otherwise come into contact with them.

You should also be aware of rings and watches. Did you ever take your watch or ring off after a hot day and see that slimy, granular stuff underneath it? That is pretty much the same stuff as under your fingernails, and just as germ ridden.

If you think that this dirt under the fingernail stuff is just more hyperbole, the US Centers for Disease Control and Prevention published proof a few years ago that a major Pseudomonas aeruginosa outbreak in a hospital was caused by the micro-organisms living under the fingernails of two nurses, one with long natural nails and another with long artificial ones. Sixteen babies died during the outbreak. If dirt under fingernails can kill 16 babies, it is certainly capable of infecting you and the people around you.

Neutralise the danger found on shoes
We are all familiar with the disinfectant-soaked mats some airports make arriving passengers walk through. This is an effective way to neutralise viruses present on the part of

the person that comes into more contact with infected surfaces than any other: the sole of the shoe.

When you consider that a single footprint-sized spot at a major airport gets stepped on over 17,000 times a day, and those 17,000 feet have just been in virtually every country on Earth in the past 24 hours, you can certainly understand the reason why a dip in a powerful disinfectant is necessary. Just the thought of all those germs being spread around where your soles can pick them up should certainly sound a warning. What if the nice gentleman standing in front of you in the queue to board a regional flight is catching a connection from Turkey, Romania or Croatia, and he had strolled around a lakeshore yesterday where his shoes picked up wild bird droppings containing H5N1? And you have just stepped in that footprint. Granted, such examples are extreme and unlikely, but the necessity to maintain sanitation on the soles of shoes is important in airports and other major transit points.

Most people don't come into contact with the floors at airports with anything but their shoes, unless their flights have been cancelled and they have no choice but to sleep on the terminal floor. However, how many times do you sit on the floor in your home, or lie down on the carpet? Your home is clean, thus you don't have to worry, right? Maybe not so right. Unless you are one of those people who have slippers at the door for guests and make them take off their shoes the instant the front door opens, every single shoe that ventures outside and then treds around your home has picked up a significant load of germs and is now spreading it around with every footstep.

But you vacuum your carpets regularly, so they are clean, right? Again, not so right. Vacuuming does very little to remove germs from carpet pile. Vacuum cleaners are designed to suck up loose, dry particulate matter, but much of the soil that contains dangerous germs is sticky and thus adheres to the pile in the carpet, often on a microscopic scale that can't readily be noticed. A professional rug shampooing with added disinfectant will do an excellent job of removing and neutralising this matter, but how many times do you get your carpets shampooed? Certainly not every time anyone walks into your home with shoes on.

It is often impractical and inconvenient to have everyone take their shoes off every time that they walk through the door, so there is another, much more convenient alternative. Take a leaf from the airport operations book: set up a shoe dip. There are various, very inexpensive ways to do this. The simplest is to take a large oven tray with a lip that is raised at least 2.5 centimetres. Then buy a cheap fibre mat (not plastic, but real, natural fibre) and cut it so that it fits snugly in the tray. Take some household disinfectant and dilute it with water according to the manufacturer's instructions. Pour enough of the solution into the tray to fill it about halfway. It might be a good idea to turn the mat upside down at this point to ensure that the fibres facing the top are well soaked. Place it just outside your door in an area sheltered from rain but where it is not practical to sidestep it in order to enter your house.

You should never use bleach in this solution as the wet shoes will leave bleached footprints on your carpet. Also you should replace the solution approximately once a week or when it is visibly dirty or cloudy.

If you're not comfortable with that, or want to really do it right, why not duplicate what the airports do? Boot mats are readily available at any agriculture or farm store, and they are deeper, sometimes over 5 centimetres. Some have a built-in serrated surface and some are even sealed within a flexible, porous 'pillowcase' that contains the disinfectant and keeps the liquid much cleaner and effective for a longer time.

However, if you are going to go down that route, then it is well worth your while to leave the household disinfectants behind and use what the pros use. Most conventional mat disinfectant solutions contain glutaraldehyde, which is a strong and nasty chemical that can cause skin rashes and more. You would be well advised to use what is arguably the best solution, which does not contain any aldehydes, and that is DuPont Virkon S. This chemical is quickly becoming the solution of choice for airports, transit areas, food processing and agricultural facilities because it is very effective and about as safe as can be to people and animals, but absolutely merciless against H5N1 viruses. Virkon S is also surprisingly affordable. A 4.5-kilogram container of the powder costs around £50/$90 but makes over 454 litres of solution, which makes it about the same price as thin bleach at the store. Don't buy the smaller packets as the price per litre increases more than tenfold. Virkon S is readily available via mail order, online sales and at many agricultural supply stores.

Virkon S is not marketed to the public, but their data safety sheets indicate there should be nothing to worry about for domestic use. Virkon S has been proven safe over years of use and, as long as you follow the manufacturer's instructions, you will find Virkon S is a superb disinfectant and possibly the best, most versatile all-round virucidal sanitiser in the world. DuPont is proud of the fact that Virkon S was even used to disinfect water during a recent Mount Everest expedition, so you can rest assured that if these mountaineers can drink it, it's safe enough to keep a mat soaked with it next to your front door.

Even with the germicidal efficiency of Virkon S, it is important to understand the mechanics of sole disinfection. The action of stepping into a shallow bath of chemicals to neutralise any germs present on the sole is clear enough. The problems occur with different shoe designs and the amount of soil on the shoe. Some shoes and boots have extremely deep treads. If you are using a homemade mat, the liquid cannot possibly soak the deeper troughs of the treads and that is where much of the contamination lies. Furthermore, if the soles have mud, faeces or anything else stuck to them, the chemical cannot disinfect that material. The shoes should be scrubbed of any visible soil before they step onto the mat.

By now you may have an image of yourself opening the door to guests, wearing yellow rubber coveralls with gloves, a respirator and a Virkon S-filled backpack tank with a spray hose to disinfect them from head to toe before they walk in. But a simple short-handled hard bristle broom by the front door, and a courteous, brief explanation of what the heck that wet mat is will not only help ensure the safety of your home environment but will also act as a conversation-starter.

Mopping your floor and washing dishes does not sterilise

Try new Mr Pure! The easy way to disinfect your floor while you damp mop! Mr Pure kills 99.9 per cent of all germs on your floor and leaves your tiles sparkling clear with a clean lemony scent. You can trust Mr Pure to keep your whole house clean, disinfected and smelling like a Mediterranean hillside!

While I don't doubt that these types of cleaners do a good job of cleaning floors, I would like to take exception to their claim of disinfectant ability.

In almost all cases when you read the label carefully you see that the claim to kill 99.9 per cent of germs is only at full strength and when left undisturbed on the surface for a minimum of ten minutes. Now, I don't know about you, but I certainly don't use undiluted cleaner on my floors and I certainly don't leave it soaking for ten minutes. The common procedure is to dilute a capful of the cleaner in a big bucket of water, mop down the floor and then rinse it with clean water. However, when you do that, you have disinfected pretty much nothing at all.

You may actually have made the germ situation worse. Damp mopping by itself can pick up germs from corners and spread them all over the floor, where they can grow even more. It can also pick up germs from the bathroom and neatly distribute them all over your kitchen floor.

We are also led to believe that a well-diluted 'miracle washing-up liquid' will leave our household items free of viruses. We have a blind trust in these washing-up liquids, especially when it says 'antibacterial' right on the label. The antiseptic qualities primarily work only when undiluted detergent is left for hours on dish sponges. The effect of such washing-up liquids when fully diluted in water on bacteria residing on dishes and glasses is negligible at best. It is patently absurd that many people now believe that all they have to do is have something even remotely soapy come into a second's contact with their greasiest, grimiest household item or surface to achieve instant sterilisation.

I see it everywhere. Many people have picked up the habit of not even rinsing off their dishes. I have been at many a spotlessly clean home where the dishes, glasses and utensils are dipped into soapy water and then placed directly on the drainer.

Dishwashing detergent and all other soaps are nothing more than surface tension diminishers. They make water a bit 'wetter' so that it can wash away particles that would normally adhere to the surfaces. Nothing more. If you don't even rinse your dishes, you're not even giving that 'wetter' water a decent chance to dislodge contaminants, which are usually microscopic and can thrive very nicely on dishes that look clean. So you dip your dishes in a diluted detergent that doesn't disinfect anything anyway, give them a quick swipe with a sponge that has several hundred thousand live germs thriving on it, don't even bother running them under clear water and let them dry to be used again later.

Viruses do not just float away into limbo at the first sign of water or soap. Very hot soapy water, so hot that you need to use gloves, may clean but only if the cups are given a thorough scrubbing and rinsing. Also, don't believe that 'antibacterial' claim on your washing-up liquid bottle. Better yet to use a modern dishwasher with the water temperature on the hottest possible setting and never turn off the 'heat dry' cycle. Viruses are irrevocably inactivated in a few seconds at 80 °C, but unfortunately many domestic dishwashers can only be set to a maximum water temperature of 65 °C (although there is always some leeway in the actual temperature so that it could be far less than this).

Fortunately if your dishwasher can maintain a minimum temperature of 60 °C for at least ten minutes at a time, it will inactivate influenza viruses such as H5N1. Even if your dishwasher can only reach 56 °C but at least can maintain this temperature for anywhere between fifteen minutes and two hours it may be effective in inactivating the influenza virus. Information on the exact temperatures achieved by each model of dishwasher is difficult to obtain, as often even the manufacturers will not make precise information available. You may want to do your homework by checking product reviews in consumer product testing publications and online. Remember that it is not sufficient for the water to enter the dishwasher at the required temperature, but it must be maintained through the wash or rinse cycle for the absolute minimum inactivation time specified.

If you're shopping for a dishwasher, try to specify a high-temperature model that uses a 'booster heater' to raise the rinse water temperature to 80 °C, hot enough to sterilise the dishes and help them dry quickly. In these models there is also a heater in the dishwasher that keeps the wash water up to temperature. Don't worry too much about the extra energy costs. It's usually more expensive to keep loading chemical sanitising agents into a low-temperature dishwasher and there is nothing quite as good for inactivating viruses on dirty dishes as a nice blast of searing 80 °C water.

One model of dishwasher that more than does the job is the Classic Duo 750. It's a commercial grade dishwasher but is almost identical in size to most household dishwashers, thus should fit wherever you could place a conventional unit. The best thing about this dishwasher is that it reaches a temperature of 85 °C, which will cremate any H5N1 or other virus. The Classic Duo 750 is quite expensive at approximately £1,500/$2,705 but one consolation is that it is somewhat in the price range of the high-end domestic dishwashers that don't reach anywhere near these temperatures. There are other commercial dishwasher models that also reach these sterilising temperatures, so if you call around to the commercial foodservice equipment suppliers in your area you may find models that suit you better. Make sure that the manufacturer will guarantee that they will reach the temperature desired. Do be aware that some plastic containers can't take these high temperatures and may warp or even melt.

Think that this is extreme? George Szatmari, professor of microbiology and immunology at the University of Montreal, says, 'Kitchens are a lot more contaminated than bathrooms. A single squeeze from a used dishcloth, dish towel or household sponge can unleash thousands, even millions, of germs onto your hands.' And Philip Tierno, director of microbiology at New York University Medical Center, says, 'If a carrot was dropped in a toilet and another dropped in the kitchen sink, I'd rather eat the carrot from the toilet.' According to Tierno, most kitchen sponges have a count of between 50,000 and 100,000 bacteria per cubic centimetre of fluid, and when raw chicken juices are left on a sponge, the bacterial count increases tenfold every hour.

Eliminating the H5N1 on your clothes

Exactly the same heat precautions apply to your laundry. There are new laundry detergents on the market that work well in cold water. They are a boon to people with delicate clothes or with non-colourfast textiles. They are also a boon to viruses. At 30 °C or 40 °C any contaminated clothes in the laundry will simply transfer their germs to all the other clothes. So even if only one piece was contaminated going in, it's likely that now all are contaminated going out.

Take your washing machine, set the water at the hottest setting and put a piece of tape over the knob. While you're at it, crank your hot water heater to the maximum setting. Be careful that you don't scald yourself by always turning on the cold-water tap first and then opening up the hot-water flow slowly until you reach the desired temperature. Having very hot water flowing into your washing machine and dishwasher will help the sanitation process also become a sterilisation one.

This may seem absurd, but you can cut down your risk of infection just by wearing white clothes. It is not the white colour of the fabric that helps minimise infection risk but the fact that white fabrics can be washed with bleach. Colourfast bleaches are not anywhere near as effective in sanitising viruses from clothing as regular thin bleach, which is sodium hypochlorite (NaOCl) at a 5.25 per cent concentration. Choose thick, resistant, white fabrics and wash them on your washing machine's hottest setting with as much bleach as the manufacturer allows and just a smidgen more. Wearing white may just help you stay alive, so leave those delicates, dark and non-colourfast fabrics in the wardrobe.

Once the laundry is washed, avoid hanging the laundry up to dry as this promotes the settlement of viruses in the textiles. Don't ever leave wet laundry sitting around, but dry it as soon as the laundry cycle is finished. Use a household dryer at the maximum temperature setting for a minimum of twenty minutes. Forget the lower settings as they are often too cool to inactivate viruses.

Remember: to inactivate viruses you need heat, lots of it, or a powerful disinfectant, with enough exposure time to kill the virus. But most people still think that soap is enough, which is symptomatic of the fact we are perpetually bombarded with advertisements telling us so. Please read this carefully:

There is no commonly available household detergent that when diluted in water and used according to manufacturer's instructions inactivates H5N1 or any other virus to any significant degree.

There are some things that do work, but they are not specifically detergents. High-quality household disinfectants are excellent virucides but, even in their case, their efficiency is severely limited through dilution with water. You should endeavour to use these disinfectants with as little dilution as feasible for the strongest virucidal action.

Generally, the best widely available substance to use for general household disinfection (next to Virkon S) is thin bleach.

Bleach is your best friend and the virus worst enemy

I've been a lifetime adherent of the wonders of bleach since I moved into my freshman dorm room at the University of California and found that in the previous semester, it had housed an entire pigsty. Every surface was visibly soiled and the room smelled like a tropical latrine. I marched down to the market in Westwood and returned with several bottles of thin bleach and rubber gloves. I spent the rest of the day drenching everything I could reach with undiluted bleach; directly out of the bottle, with no water in sight. My roommate was convinced that my skin and the rest of the room would bubble up and melt upon contact with the bleach, but that didn't happen. What did happen was that everything was sparkling clear, fully disinfected, had that clean bleach smell and it was a pleasure to live there.

One of the most important things I learned at UCLA in my freshman year was that bleach is incredibly effective and is nowhere near as corrosive or dangerous as people think. I drop a couple of capfuls of thin bleach in my bathwater before jumping in. I've been doing that for more than a quarter of a century and I have never had any ill effects from it.

During a flu pandemic your skin can come into contact with thousands of active viruses in the environment. It is a traditional home remedy to bathe in a weak bleach solution to kill germs on your skin. The dosage should not exceed 120 millilitres of common household bleach to a full conventional bathtub. Don't worry about this concentration hurting your skin. It's really not much more than a well-chlorinated swimming pool. A typical bathtub contains 120 litres, thus the dilution is 1,000 to 1. Since bleach is the active ingredient sodium hypochlorite (NaOCl) already diluted 20 to 1, your bath contains only 1 part NaOCl to 20,000 parts water. At this concentration, it is safe enough to drink, thus should certainly not harm your skin. After the bath, more sensitive individuals can use a skin lotion to prevent dryness or chapping, but I have never known that to occur.

For those unwilling to bathe in even a diluted bleach solution, weak concentrations of hydrogen peroxide (60 millilitres per tub) or even high concentrations of salt (2 kilograms per tub) are acceptable alternatives. Any water treatment chemical used in hot tubs and spas will work as a reasonably effective virucidal bath. The people who shun chlorine and bromine can use colloidal silver, ionised copper, etc. Check with your local spa supply store for its effective solutions. They are tested to be safe and can be used in your bath just as easily as in a hot tub or spa.

Rubbing Alcohol (usually 70 per cent isopropyl alcohol) is readily available, very inexpensive and quite effective if liberally applied with a sponge to the entire body. If you do that after a shower you will feel refreshed as the alcohol evaporates and cools off your body. It's quite bracing and extremely virucidal.

The more common use for bleach is not bathing but for the disinfection of household surfaces. I don't recommend that you use undiluted bleach on your floors, but I do recommend that you use a stronger dilution than is normally recommended. Most sources will recommend that you dilute 1 part bleach to 100 parts water. That is an effective dilution, but if you want to rest a bit more assured of virucidal efficiency, go to 1 part bleach to 20 parts really hot water. There isn't a virus around that can survive a good splash of that mixture. Make sure that you thoroughly rinse the floor with plenty of fresh clean water afterwards and you'll have a floor that you can literally eat off.

Most linoleum or ceramic tiles are wonderfully resistant to bleach, but there are a few floor types that will be damaged by it, such as hardwood flooring. In those cases, note that Virkon S has been tested on porous surfaces such as wood and it works admirably. That makes it a perfect choice for disinfecting wooden floors, countertops, even wooden cutting boards that get splintery after too much bleach. Most disinfectants are ineffective on porous surfaces such as wood, but not Virkon S – another reason why it's a good choice for much of your household disinfection, even though DuPont has specifically not marketed the product for household use.

Something else that works wonders on household items is good old boiling water. It works a charm to sterilise everything that it touches. By far the best way to sanitise dishes and cutlery is to run them through the dishwasher then place them in the sink and cover them in rolling boiling water, right off the stove. No matter how hot or cool your dishwasher water may have been, that will wipe out any viruses hitching a ride.

Kashering: What the Jews knew 6,000 years ago that we ve recently discovered

The act of kashering or making a kitchen kosher dates back several millennia. It is still practised with the same fervour of thousands of years ago in most modern Jewish homes. Given the fact that the Western world has only really understood the nature of microbes over the last century, it is remarkable that an ancient society would incorporate into their religion the act of sterilising everything in their kitchens in a very modern and effective manner.

The methods of kashering include the following:

- *Libun Gamur*, which means 'complete purification'. This means heating a pan or grill until it is red hot. A conventional oven does not reach the temperatures needed to heat pans until they are red hot and this is a procedure that is usually performed by a rabbi with a blowtorch. I don't recommend taking an oxyacetylene to your skillets, so let's move on.
- *Libun Kal*, which means 'simple purification'. This is the process of heating metal pots, pans, grills, etc hot enough that a broom straw touching the other side of it immediately scorches. You can substitute a bit of crumpled newspaper. Ovens that have a self-cleaning cycle arrive at this temperature. It's an excellent method of sterilising any metal container or implement. Just pop it

into the self-cleaning oven and start the cycle. Beware that if there are any handles or other parts made of anything but metal they will quickly melt or could even be set on fire.

- *Hag'alah*, which means 'scouring' or 'scalding', is used for items such as pots or cutlery by setting them in a large pot of boiling water.
- *Irui*, which means 'infusion', is most often used for countertops and sinks. Boiling water right off the stove is poured all over them. Beware that some countertop veneers may come unglued under boiling water. Ensure that your countertop can survive this process before you do it.

Everything in a kosher kitchen has to be kashered. There are long, formal, comprehensive lists of how to properly kasher almost anything from microwave ovens to water coolers. These lists are readily available on the internet by just typing 'kashering' on any search engine, or you could drop in at your local synagogue. The rabbi should be more than happy to assist you. In virtually every case the procedures indicated adhere to good, modern sterilising practice and can be used in the bathroom as well as the kitchen. A freshly kashered kitchen or bathroom is about as germ-free an environment as can legitimately be achieved outside a negative-pressure laboratory clean room.

Most surgical face masks are ineffective: Where to buy the ones that work

We have all seen respirator masks. Every time we watch a a hospital drama show on television we see the doctors and nurses wearing them. We have also seen scenes of people in Asia wearing them around town when they don't want to become infected or are already contagious and don't wish to infect others.

Respirators are used to reduce the risk of inhaling germs. They do so by filtering the air you breathe and trapping contaminants before they get to you. There are many different types of respirators, and most of them are quite ineffective. The problem is not in the filtering, but in the fit. Most respirators do not form an effective seal around the edge where the mask touches your skin. The airflow into your nose and mouth then takes a detour around the mask, through those gaps and into you, obviating the efficiency of the most well-designed filter.

No filter short of a NASA spacesuit or a biohazard lab-suit (Level four and up) will provide 100 per cent protection against H5N1. But if you have chosen to wear a respirator as part of your self-protection process then you should learn which models are the most effective.

There are several major types of disposable particulate respirators used in viral contagion situations. They are rated according to the percentage of airborne particles that they will filter out during a 'worst case' scenario, so the actual real world performance should be better yet.

Respirators that filter out at least 95 per cent of airborne particles receive a '95' rating. Those that filter out a minimum of 99 per cent receive a '99' rating. And those that filter at least 99.97 per cent (essentially 100 per cent) receive a '100' rating. These types of respirators are rated as N, R, or P for protection against oils. This rating is important because some oils can degrade the efficiency of the filter. That is especially important in situations where you can come into contact with oil, during cooking, when working in a garage, etc. Respirators are rated 'N' if they are not resistant to oil, 'R' if somewhat resistant to oil, and

'P' if strongly resistant (virtually oil proof). Therefore that designates a total of nine types of respirator:

N-95, N-99, N-100
R-95, R-99, R-100
P-95, P-99, P-100

Which level of protection is best for you? The 99s and 100s cost a bit more than the 95s, but the cost is rather negligible. The N, R and P ratings are a bit different. Unless I was planning on deep-frying potatoes or doing automotive oil changes all day, I'd choose the N for everyday use.

The US National Institute for Occupational Safety and Health (NIOSH) applies very high standards to test and approve respirators. NIOSH-approved disposable respirators are marked with the manufacturer's name, the part number, the protection provided by the filter (such as N-95) and 'NIOSH'. This information is printed on the face piece, exhalation valve cover or head straps. Look for these marks to ensure that you are getting a properly tested and approved respirator. There are other standards institutes in various nations that also approve respirators with varying standards, but I recommend looking for the NIOSH label.

The best respirator is not going to filter out much of anything unless it is fitted correctly. These nine types of respirator have similar fit characteristics, so they can all be considered pretty well the same when it comes to fitting your face. Follow the instructions that come with the mask very carefully to make sure that you are fitting the mask correctly. A common mistake is that people fit the straps of their mask over the sides of their glasses or goggles, which reduces the snugness of the respirator's fit on your face and thus its efficiency. Take any glasses or goggles off first, fit the mask, then put them back on over the straps.

Some of these respirators are designed with an exhalation valve. The valve is useful as it reduces warmth and moisture that can build up inside the mask. When you breathe out, the valve opens to release the exhaled air and then snaps shut during inhalation so that inhaled air has to pass through the filter.

The reason not all respirators have these valves is that they make the protection one-way only. A respirator without a valve protects against viruses coming from the outside world into you as well as from you to the outside world. When you add a valve, the respirator is as effective at keeping the viruses from the outside world from getting into you, but does not stop viruses from your body potentially infecting others.

Whichever type you decide to use, it is important to note that respirators are to be considered strictly disposable. Whenever they are worn in an environment that can be considered even remotely contagious, they have to be thrown away, with care being taken to never touch the outside of the respirator where the trapped particles lie. You must give your hands a thorough wash immediately afterwards. The best thing to do with discarded respirators if you don't have access to hospital-level contagious waste disposal is to burn them. There are procedures to reuse respirators but, if I was wearing them, I'd stock up with a whole bunch of them and only use each one once.

There is, however, one 'small' problem with these types of respirators. The filters have a 'grille opening' of 0.3 microns, which will stop almost everything larger than that, but have virtually no effect on anything smaller. Since H5N1 is approximately 0.1 micron, it will just flow right through the filter. Only if some H5N1 viruses are attached to larger particles of dust or water droplets will the filters have any effect. Fortunately that is the case most of the time, but there are still some rogue loner viruses around. Think of the filter as your home's front door. You can walk through it with no problem, but it's not wide enough to drive your car through it. Therefore, the filter doesn't do much for the tiny H5N1 virus, unless it's riding on a much larger 'car type' particle that can't fit through the front door.

Well, it does turn out that many H5N1 viruses are piggy-backing on other particles, water, and all sorts of things that are larger than 0.3 microns and that is why NIOSH and other agencies consider filtering down to this level perfectly adequate. But the niggling fact remains that the H5N1 virus is much, much smaller than this. A dozen H5N1 viruses clustered into a ball could easily pass through a single 0.3-micron opening without touching the sides.

Since we're trying to find the most effective methods of keeping as safe as possible, it is well worth considering the NanoMask by Emergency Filtration Technology. The NanoMask has not yet been tested by NIOSH at the time of writing, but there is some believable science behind it that suggests their claim to filter out 0.027 micron particles is to be taken legitimately. When it comes to the NanoMask, those H5N1 viruses that could dance like a chorus line through the 0.3-micron holes will find themselves in the position of an overweight man trying to squeeze in through the door of his chihuahua's kennel.

While we're at it, why not go all the way and wear eye protection as well? The eyes are a direct conduit for infection so they need to be protected as well. A snug-fitting set of goggles that create an airtight seal are best. There are also full facemask respirators that look like welding visors with hoses to backpacks, but that is getting a bit too far out there even for my tastes. If you're in an environment that is *that* contagious, then you'd be best to turn tail and run away.

Destroy the thousands of germs on a common home/office appliance

In the days before universal mobile phones, I was waiting to use what seemed to be the only public telephone in a town square near Ensenada, Mexico. The man who was using the phone had a monstrously nasty cold and he would sneeze and snort and cough with virtually every sentence. After a few minutes of this, I decided that my important telephone call was not that important and just walked away. By the time he had finished his call, that telephone handset would have been completely coated in the man's viruses. The only way I was going to use it would be if I could first dunk it in a bucket of bleach, but I don't think that the Mexican Telephone Company would be too happy with me if I did that.

A similar situation presented itself years later when I was waiting at a very busy internet café in London for an open terminal. Finally one became available but it had been used by a young man who kept wiping his runny nose with his hands while continuing to type. Once again, I decided that I didn't need to check my email that badly.

But what can you do in those situations? Sensitive electronics cannot be subjected to disinfectant chemicals. They will short out and it could start a fire. Alcohol is an excellent disinfectant and can be used in some cases on electronics but not always. One solution that prevents applying any liquid to electronics is found in a simple and inexpensive device that resembles a fluorescent blacklight flashlight with the tube shining out of the side instead of the end. Simply turn on the light and wave it about 5 centimetres over the keyboard, mouse, phone or other equipment for a few seconds for a surprisingly effective sanitisation.

The key to this action is ultraviolet (UV) light. UV is an invisible light that has a frequency below that of visible light. The visible spectrum stretches from approximately 780 to 400 nanometres. A nanometre is one billionth of a metre. There are three bands of UV light, starting at the UV-A from 400 nanometres then going onto UV-B from 315 nanometres. These bands are generally known as the 'suntanning' frequencies. The UV light that has germicidal effect is UV-C. This particular wavelength finds its peak effectiveness in inactivating viruses and bacteria at 254 nanometres.

When a virus is subjected to UV-C the light passes right through it, disrupting the molecular bonds that hold its DNA (or RNA) together. This rupturing leaves the virus unable to replicate and it becomes fully inactive moments later.

These types of flashlights have a UV-C bulb incorporated within them. They are used by mineral collectors for identifying glowing elements and for other forensic uses. All you need to do is carry one with you everywhere you go. When you need to touch a surface that has likely been contaminated, just point the flashlight tube close towards the surface, turn it on, wave it around for a couple of seconds and then rest assured that any germ on that surface has just been delivered a lethal dose of UV radiation.

As in the case of all UV-C lighting, you have to exercise caution. You don't want to spend any time at all being irradiated by UV-C light as it can affect your eyes. The first sign is that it may feel as if there is sand in your eyes.

It can also cause skin effects not too unlike a nasty sunburn. UV-C light is very dangerous and you should always take the precautions recommended by the bulb manufacturer. Don't look at the light or point it towards yourself or anyone else, and practise holding the flashlight when it's off so that your fingers aren't exposed to the bulb. Don't keep the light on for more than a few seconds at a time because that's all the time it needs to deliver its effective disinfectant action.

These little flashlights also have another magical use. If you're confronted with water that you're concerned might be contaminated with bacteria or viruses, all you need to do is to pour the water into a clean, clear glass (make sure that it's made of transparent glass and not plastic), then shine the flashlight onto it for a couple of seconds. Give the glass a quarter turn. Another couple of seconds of zapping. Repeat this until you've delivered light energy to each quarter turn of the glass and then drink away. This UV light will have no effect on chemicals within the glass (so if the water is poisoned, it's not going to help) and will not kill any significant waterborne parasites. But if you're concerned about bacterial or viral contamination in that water, you can rest assured that now it's perfectly safe to drink. You may find, however, that sterilising tablets are better suited to this task.

Sanitise your bathroom by just changing a light fixture

There is an easy to install and very affordable alternative that has a marked level of efficiency in inactivating H5N1 and other viruses and bacteria by safely exposing them to UV germicidal light in any room. It's called the UV Upper Room option.

UV Upper Room basically looks like a standard fluorescent light fixture but it's mounted upside down so that it is shining up not down. The way it works is that the regular airflow through your room causes constant mixing, thus the air is always circulating. This circulation is even more marked in the winter months because warm air from the heating system rises to the top of the room, creating a constant vertical slowly spinning vortex. As the air flows past the UV system, the viruses and bacteria in the air are subjected to the UV light and inactivated. That's why it is important to get a significant amount of air flowing past the UV fixture. The more airflow, the more germs get zapped. UV Upper Room systems are most effective when the heat source from the room comes from as far down as possible, such as baseboard heating, however, the airflow 'vortex' in the room can also be increased by operating a small fan in the room, pointing straight up.

There are other factors to consider. Distance from the UV light source to the germ to be killed decreases by approximately the square of the distance from the lamp. At 2.5 centimetres from the lamp it's delivering one 'unit' of zapping power, but if you move 5 centimetres from the lamp, the power has dropped to 1/4. When you're 20 centimetres away it's gone down all the way to 1/64. So it's always advisable to make sure that the air containing your nasties is brought as close to the lamp as feasible for maximum zapping action.

UV lamps vary widely in radiating power as there are many different designs and specifications. A little homework and a quick look at the Resources section at the end of this book will help you choose the best fit for your system. And remember that you can always add more lamps for more power.

The time that the germ is subjected to the UV light is also important. The longer it's exposed, the more effective the disinfection. UV Upper Room fixtures are very safe since they are designed in such a way that UV energy doesn't significantly leak into the room at 'people' level.

There are some installations where the UV light points down into the room. These installations are claimed to be effective in sanitising the surfaces of the room, such as toilets and sinks. However, generally speaking, the risk you take for your eyes and skin is not worth the installation of these units. Remember the inverse square law we discussed earlier. From a ceiling height, a germ on a toilet seat would be receiving less than 1/1,000th the zapping energy it would receive if it were only 2.5 centimetres away from the lamp. To combat this and to provide eye and skin safety, some of these installations are set up so that they are wired into the bathroom light switch. When you turn the main light on, the UV light goes off. Then when you leave and turn the main light on, the UV light goes on. Since your bathroom is typically used about an hour a day, that leaves the other 23 hours for the UV light to work its magic. This is not a recommended technique, however. It's not very safe as sometimes you go into your bathroom without the light on, subjecting yourself to UV. Also, prolonged exposure to UV light can break down some of the plastics in the bathroom such as toilet seats and linoleum. It's much better to go with a professionally designed UV Upper Room option, especially if you can increase the airflow with a strategically mounted fan.

Inactivating H5N1 viruses with light

The popular term 'Sick Building Syndrome' refers to a dangerous situation when bacterial and viral contamination reaches critical levels in heating and air conditioning (HVAC) equipment and systems. In these cases, the inhabitants or workers in these buildings can have symptoms ranging from nausea to chronic fatigue. One of the remedies developed to sanitise the air passing through these HVAC systems is UV air disinfection.

HVAC UV can only be installed in buildings that have forced air systems. If a building is fitted with hot water radiators then there are usually no ducts to fit the UV system within. A typical HVAC UV system installation in a forced air system building would see the UV unit about 30 centimetres down the air stream from the system's coil to maximise the germicidal effect of the light on that critical component. It is sometimes also placed in the return air duct, thereby sanitising the volume of air entering the HVAC system. The best results are obtained when both placements are installed.

HVAC UV systems are meant to be professionally installed and maintained. The lamps radiate very powerful levels of light that are not intended for human exposure. Lamps should be replaced approximately every year as their output drops as they age.

HVAC UV is a powerful tool against airborne H5N1. The virus is quite fragile in the air and the strong irradiation with UV light is extremely effective in inactivating it. A dream system for a hypothetical home of approximately 93 square metres would be a properly installed UV system in the forced air HVAC ducts and near the coil and then three air purifiers, such as the Plasmacluster 60 model, equally spaced throughout the house. The cost of such a system would perhaps not be prohibitive, as it could be implemented at a cost of around £2,000/$3,600, fully installed, which these days is not a huge amount to pay for a home health improvement of this magnitude. With the UV and ions working in unison, you could be assured that your home's air would be highly disinfected. Although it would be impossible to guarantee that the interior air would be 100 per cent H5N1-free, the amount of virus in the internal residential environment would be diminished significantly.

Where to buy an air-cleaning device

There is only one commercially available air purifier that has a reasonable claim to significantly and effectively inactivate H5N1 in the air. It is the Plasmacluster, manufactured by Sharp and developed by Professor John Oxford of the University of London. It uses air filtration combined with ion bombardment and in clinical tests conducted by the manufacturer it has been shown to inactivate more than 99 per cent of H5N1 viruses in the air. Note that this is not peer-reviewed clinical testing published in a leading medical journal, so some issue can be taken with it. Regardless, by the evidence offered it seems to present a level of H5N1 disinfection in air that other air purifiers can't match.

A Plasmacluster is a rather large floor-standing unit that resembles a flattened freestanding air conditioner or humidifier. Inside the Plasmacluster there is an ion generator that uses an alternating plasma discharge to split some of the water molecules in the air into hydrogen and oxygen ions by shooting them with a strong electric current and oppositely charging them. Now these ions have a positive and negative charge and they are attracted to particles in the air by their electrical charge. The positive hydrogen ions are attracted to the negatively charged particles, and the negative oxygen ions are attracted to the positively charged particles. These positive and negative ions surround the airborne particle and react to form a substance called hydroxyl.

This hydroxyl has an interesting effect on viruses. It surrounds them and rips hydrogen atoms away from their surface. The hydroxyl is a radical, thus is highly unstable. In order to stabilise itself, it will steal one hydrogen atom from any airborne particle it comes into contact with. When the particle is a germ such as a virus, this has the effect of inactivating the virus and returning the hydroxyl to droplets of water. The process takes only a fraction of a second thus there is no danger of coming into contact with hydroxyl radicals (which have been linked to DNA damage). The ions are not allowed to accumulate on a surface, so cannot not reach a high enough density to form hydroxyl. When these positive and negative ions come in contact with our skin, the much stronger electrical field generated by our bodies swiftly neutralises them without forming hydroxyl. The hydroxyl action generated by the Plasmacluster's positive and negative ions is therefore only effective on microscopic airborne germs.

The Plasmacluster continually sprays out these positive and negative ions to inactivate airborne germs and combines it with a multiple filter system including a high-efficiency particulate (HEPA) to be even more effective against most airborne germs. Unfortunately the HEPA filter has the same 0.3-micron grille opening as the N-95 respirators discussed earlier. Thus, the Plasmacluster's ion effect is the truly significant function it has against H5N1 as the filter can't effectively stop lone viruses.

The UV options and the Plasmacluster are not iron-clad 100 per cent effective solutions to disinfecting the air in your environment and keeping it H5N1-free. Nothing can do that. You have to determine for yourself if the measure of virucidal action they provide is worth the cost.

Common sense is your best friend

As with many other tips in this book, these are rarely specific only to H5N1. They are general warnings of practices that transmit other germs and may transmit H5N1 or suggestions for preventing infection in general that should be effective against H5N1. Regardless, it is imperative to stay healthy and free from as many infections as possible in times of pandemic, so you should endeavour to follow as many of these tips as you can reasonably incorporate into your lifestyle.

- If your country has a health advice line, get the number and keep it to hand. These numbers are usually very easy to find by dialling directory assistance or checking the Yellow Pages. In the UK the NHS Direct number is 08454647. The number in New Zealand is 0800-611116. In some countries health information is dispensed by individual states or provinces. In Australia, for example, the ACT's number is 132281, and there are different ones for each state. These information services are invaluable resources for all forms of health questions and you should make ample use of this service to help identify symptoms or get other health and prevention advice. Don't wait until the pandemic hits as the phone lines may be jammed. Draw up a list of questions you require clarifications on, and call them today.

- Inhalation and ingestion are the two main ways for H5N1 to enter your body. Consider a sneezing or coughing individual as a clear biohazard. Stay away from their sneezing spray or coughing radius. Cover your own mouth and nose when you cough or sneeze to prevent others becoming infected and then dispose of the tissue immediately. Ingestion does not mean eating the virus. It refers to touching your eyes, mouth or nose with hands that have come into contact with H5N1. You must consider your hands to be an extremely effective contagion mechanism, which must be kept scrupulously clean and sanitised.

- Prolonged exposure to being cold and wet lowers your resistance and increases your risk of infection. Avoid spending time outside in inclement weather. There are many people who won't venture to the corner store if it's cold or wet, yet will think nothing of watching a football match in freezing rain. Stay inside and watch it on the telly.

- If you have to go outside in bad weather, take precautions to stay warm and dry. Wear a warm coat and raingear over it. Make sure you have a hood and keep it up over your head to keep water from seeping down the back of your neck. Umbrellas are ineffective if there is even a mild wind, so don't count on them to keep you dry. Keep your hands, feet and especially the top of your head warm. In cold weather most of your heat loss is through your skull. Wear insulated headwear. If you get wet underneath your rainwear, go inside and dry off, even if it has to be in a public toilet or the changing room of a department store.

What You Can Do Now

- Smoking and alcohol can impair your resistance. Alcohol suppresses the immune system and there is clinical proof of the link between alcoholism and severe infections. Smoking injures the respiratory tract, slows the cilia (which push contaminants out of your lungs) and increases flu susceptibility. That applies to second-hand smoke as well. You can be in severe danger even if a cigarette has never touched your lips. If people around you are smoking, tell them to go outside. If you work in a job where you are surrounded by smokers, get another job. Don't think that pipe or cigar smoke is somehow better for you than cigarettes. All tobacco smoke is the same.

- Kissing is a very efficient way to transmit flu. Mucous membrane to mucous membrane contact is a virus autobahn. Remember that your partner may be contagious days before showing any symptoms. Put the mistletoe away and cool your amorous advances. Sleeping in the same room with a sick spouse is also ill-advised. The guest bedroom or sofa is advised for the duration.

- If you are not getting a minimum of seven or, better yet, eight hours of sleep a night, do whatever necessary to do so. Go to bed earlier, drink a hot toddy, or even resort to sleeping medication. If your spouse's snoring keeps you awake, exile them to the sofa.

- Don't get tired or run-down. During a pandemic is not the time to overwork, stress out or engage in strenuous activities. If something is stressing you out, get away from it. That includes work issues.

Cut down on your overtime, don't take on extra work, and if someone proposes a big new project or task to qualify you for that long-awaited promotion, inform them that you don't mind waiting a bit longer.

- Regular light exercise is best. Don't go to the gym and work yourself into a lather or go running until you go 'through the wall'. Aerobics and aquarobics are recommended for their smooth, steady actions. Keep your exercise at least 10 per cent below your target heart rate until the pandemic is well past.

- H5N1 can't last too long out in the environment but other germs can linger on wet toothbrush bristles, making it easy to reinfect yourself day after day. Buy a large supply of toothbrushes and toss them away regularly. Don't let anyone ever touch your toothbrush.

- Clean, clean and clean some more. The bottom of some people's toasters is suitable for archaeological digs. Throw away the mouldy crumbs and disinfect the tray regularly. Keep pantries, cupboards, shelves and any food storage areas scrupulously clean. Defrost your refrigerator and freezer regularly and clean them completely. Do you have any idea what is growing underneath your fridge, stove and other large household appliances? Move them and clean the filthy mess underneath. The same goes for large furniture. Move it all out of the way and vacuum, sweep or mop underneath. Turn your mattress over and spray it with a good-quality household disinfectant. A good shot of insecticide wouldn't hurt either. Some people I know stick a couple of pet flea collars inside the mattress itself and they claim it works wonders in keeping the mites down. Change the collars every two months and don't let them come into contact with your skin. Put your bedding, duvets and pillows into the washing machine regularly. If your pillow or duvet can't be laundered, throw it away and buy one that can.

- If the males in your household insist on spraying urine all around the toilet, force them to sit down. Some uncircumcised men can't help but have their urine go off in multiple directions as their foreskins interfere with the stream. Have them pull back their foreskin when they urinate, but the best way is always to have a seat.

- Avoid team sports, contact with crowds and busy restaurants. If you have to go shopping try the 24-hour supermarket between midnight and 8 am, when they are nearly deserted. If you want to shop on the high street, try it first thing in the morning as soon as the stores open. You'll face far fewer crowds and you'll find your shopping is faster and more pleasant.

- Different cultures have different 'comfort spheres'. Many Nordic people will keep a fair distance from you when speaking and are uncomfortable if you get too close. Many southern people like to almost touch noses with you. I once knew a Mexican gentleman who would only speak to you if he could put his hands on your shoulders. Adopt the Nordic attitude, regardless of your heritage; it will help minimise infection.

- Quit your bad habits. Stop biting your nails, as the germs hiding beneath them can easily infect you through your mouth. If you chew tobacco then put it away. If you're into dangerous extreme sports, start watching them on television instead of participating. You don't need to risk any undue hospital visits during a pandemic.

- Designate at least one rubbish bin in your house a 'no touch' container. Make sure that it has a snugly fitting pivoting lid and use it for the disposal of anything that could even remotely be contagious. Treat the bag as biohazardous material: buy the thickest and strongest bags available; only touch it with rubber gloves; seal it with a twist or nylon tie; and beware when you are taking it out. Bags leak or rupture and the contents can be infectious, especially the ones from 'no touch' containers. Always wear rubber gloves and keep your arm out straight so that the bag is as far from your body as possible. If your clothes become stained from rubbish, change them immediately. Always wash the entire container and lid with hot soapy water and diluted bleach every time you change the bag.

- Change your lifestyle. Don't go out clubbing where you'll be spending the night in close proximity to 10,000 strangers. If you take narcotics, check into a rehab centre. Never perform oral sex without a mouth dam or condom. Never perform anal or vaginal sex without a condom. Be aware that most condoms are designed for cart-horses and have no real-world relation to the size of the average penis. Men, check the sizes on the sides of the boxes and buy the smallest one available. Check online and specialty condom sources for even smaller sizes. The average erect penis is well under 15.2 centimetres long and in some races under 12.7 centimetres so don't think you are abnormally tiny. Unless you are one of the fortunate few, the condom will be too large and will not fit snugly enough around the base of your penis to keep all the contents safely inside. Pull out immediately after ejaculating and don't lose your erection while still wearing your condom. Dispose of the condom and any other paraphernalia in a 'no touch' container. Carefully clean any vibrators and sex toys with rubbing alcohol after every use. Treat all genital and other bodily fluids as contagious and if you come into contact with them, wash thoroughly immediately. Lesbian sex is contagious as well and the same precautions should be taken as with sex involving males. Avoid sexual contact during menstruation due to the larger amounts of fluids from the female. Try monogamy, or turn to cyber sex. H5N1 is not a sexually transmitted disease per se as it can be transmitted just as easily during a casual kiss or a handshake as through full intercourse. Remember that during times of pandemic you certainly don't want to be down with another infection that may weaken your system and allow H5N1 to take a foothold where one might ordinarily not be present.

- Practise planned parenthood. Avoid pregnancy at all costs until the pandemic has passed. Pregnant women and their foetuses could be in greater danger from H5N1.

- Bring grandma or grandpa home. A care home is a prime breeding ground for infections. Your elderly relatives are much better off in your own home for the duration. You will all stay healthier that way as when you visit them at the care home you can easily become infected.
- Don't send kids off on school field trips or holidays. Consider home tutoring (check with your educational authority to see if it's legal in your area) to keep your kids out of the contagious arena that schools have no choice but to be.
- With skyrocketing energy prices, people are battening down and weather-stripping their homes so that not a single molecule of expensively warmed air can escape. That is good economy and bad practice. You have to air out your house regularly as the stale air can harbour a remarkable amount of germs. Many people, especially in urban settings, are afraid of keeping windows open for fear of burglaries. Some new windows allow you to keep them securely locked but still have them cracked open by a tiny bit to let airflow in as they have a second locking flange a bit further out. I have them in my house and heartily recommend them. Besides, there is a radioactive gas called radon that can seep into your house from underground and if you don't air out your house regularly, it can be extremely dangerous.
- If you have a health question, call your doctor or surgery instead of setting an appointment. Unless you require treatment, avoid visits to hospitals, surgeries, pharmacies, health clinics and anywhere else that sick people congregate. Remember to

stay healthy from unrelated ailments. If you have an abscessed tooth, swollen tonsils, constipation or any other niggling health problem you've been putting off treating, do it now.

- Kids are germ magnets. Almost everything about a child's lifestyle is an infection opportunity waiting to happen. Supervise your children to keep them off the floor. Don't let them roll around outside on the lawn or pavement. Keep toys scrupulously clean. Some younger children constantly put toys in their mouths thus they cannot be bleached. Try scrubbing them with hot soapy water or use one of those UV-C devices I discussed earlier as they leave no residues behind that can harm children. Dirty nappies are incredible germ reservoirs. Dispose of them carefully in a 'no touch' container and always wash your hands thoroughly afterwards.

- Keep your pets indoors for the duration of the pandemic. They will adapt quite nicely to the indoor life and learn to love it. Dogs and cats that run around outside can bring in a plethora of germs. They can bring in on their paws H5N1-infected bird droppings or, even worse, an infected bird. Dogs can be litter trained like cats, however, I'd be concerned if I owned a dog the size of a Great Dane. Consider dirty litter as a complete biohazard and dispose of it carefully in your 'no touch' container. Pregnant women and small children should always keep far away from animal waste.

- Never use a handkerchief for any reason. Replace them with disposable tissues and make sure that you dispose of them in 'no touch' containers. If you are silly enough to go outside without a supply of disposable tissues, sneeze or cough in the crook of your elbow, not in your hand.

- Replace the hand towels in your bathroom and kitchen with paper towels. Dispose of them in a 'no touch' container as well.

- Don't ever re-wear clothing unless it's been thoroughly and properly laundered. Don't pick your day's clothes out of the dirty clothes hamper or off the floor. Treat any clothes that have come into contact with infectious individuals as bio-hazards. Keep them separate and launder them immediately in the hottest water with bleach if possible. Dispose of them otherwise. Don't forget to sanitise purses, bags, belts, jewellery and other accessories.

- When you sit on a toilet, whether public or even in your own home, don't let your trousers or skirt touch the floor. Hold them up with one hand if you have to, or better yet, take them off completely and hang them on a hook.

- Put off throwing or attending parties or community gatherings until the pandemic is over. Try to avoid letting people other than your family into your home. Every person that walks in is a potential contagion risk even if you keep your house spotless and sanitised.

- If you do have to have a gathering, don't stack coats, especially on your bed. When you hang coats and jackets in your foyer closet keep them separate and make sure that they don't touch each other. You may be well advised to hang plastic sheeting from every other hanger and only place the coats between the sheeted hangers.

- Put off any travel whether holiday or business. Other countries may have much less rigorous infection control standards. Besides, can you think of a more infectious place to sit for several hours than a train or aeroplane? Avoid cruises completely. They can turn to floating sealed containers of infection.

- Save your money. Keep as much money in secure savings as you can. You may have to take extended time off work or even lose your job and your income may suffer. Have a substantial overdraft agreement with your bank or have several credit cards with plenty of credit limit left on them. Sign up for the schemes where you pay a bit of money every month and receive coverage of your credit card and other payments if you get ill.

- This seems macabre, but place large life insurance policies on everyone in your family, including yourself. The short term and long term costs of losing a family member are incalculable.

- Don't share anything with anybody: dishes, cutlery, cups, glasses, towels, bedding or anything else.

- Beware of restaurant cutlery and dishes. Be especially careful of cups in cafés. If they look even remotely soiled, don't touch them and ask for a clean one. It's a good practice to carefully wipe with a paper napkin one spot of the cup and drink from that part only.

- Keep yourself well hydrated to help keep infection at bay. Drink a minimum of eight 237-millilitre glasses of water a day. Beer, coffee and tea do not contribute to this total as they can be diuretics. If you can't stand plain water, try the lightly fruity 'designer waters' or soft drinks. Make sure that they are sugar-free, as sugared drinks also do not contribute to the eight glasses a day total. Always choose caffeine-free drinks for better hydration. Don't believe the claims of 'superhydration' by expensive 'sports drinks'. There is nothing better for your body than fresh, cool, clean water.

- A sauna is a surprisingly effective way to rid your skin of viruses. It will have to be a real sauna where the temperature exceeds 77 °C, which is quite hot but tolerable. Any H5N1 virus on your skin cannot survive in these temperatures, and although the efficiency is attenuated by the cooling effect of your perspiration, that can be minimised by regular towelling off. The higher you sit in a sauna, the hotter it will be, as hot air rises. Don't stay in for more than 15 minutes, and leave immediately if you feel faint or nauseous. Never fall asleep in a sauna. Drink lots of fluids inside and outside, but beware that a bottle of cool water will soon become scalding. If you have to do it the Finnish way and be naked, sit on a clean towel, but don't join your more foolhardy friends in jumping into a frozen lake as a cool shower will do nicely. Also you don't have to go to extremes and sit in saunas of 120 °C or more. These are temperatures of 20 °C above the boiling point of water. Humans simply are not suited to these temperatures. You are trying to kill viruses, not turn yourself into a boiled sausage.

What You Can Do Now

- I don't know why this has to be mentioned as it seems common sense to me, but eat well. Use the five-a-day plan or the food pyramid, or anything else you want, but keep yourself in good nutritional status. This is not the time to diet, no matter if it's Atkins, GI, South Beach, Low-Cal, The Zone or anything else. If you gain a bit you can always take it off after the pandemic has passed. Beware of crackpots and quacks that claim that eating this, that or the other thing will keep you safe from flu. A balanced diet with regular exercise is always the best.
- This is another common sense one that I can't believe has to be mentioned, but flush the toilet after every use.
- Look on eBay to find a used NASA spacesuit in good condition and wear it 24/7 through the pandemic. If you can afford it, pay £20/$36 million to go live on the International Space Station for the duration. (OK, I'm only joking about these ones!)
- Remember your mantra: Don't panic. Don't panic. Don't panic. Now repeat your mantra: Don't panic. Don't panic. Don't panic . . .

CHAPTER 6

Don't Eat H5N1

How to keep from bringing home flu in your grocery bag

Here are some good tips to follow to keep your food supply from infecting you with H5N1. Since much food safety is indicated to prevent a wide variety of germ-borne contamination, few of these are specific to H5N1, but they are an excellent way to ensure that H5N1 or other viruses and bacteria don't infect you through your groceries. Note that H5N1 in a pandemic situation would primarily be transmitted through inhalation and ingestion by contact of hands to the eyes and mouth. The actual ingestion of food infected with H5N1 would account for a very small percentage of human infections.

- Almost a third of all people thaw frozen poultry or meat on the kitchen counter, in the oven or under hot water in the sink. Frozen meats should always be thawed or marinated in a refrigerator set below 4 °C. Check your fridge temperature with an accurate thermometer. More than a third of all fridges are much warmer than 4 °C and thus unsafe. Freezers must be set to below -1 °C and preferably far below that. H5N1 cannot replicate in processed poultry but lots of other nasties can hide in there.

- Four out of five cooks believe that it's necessary to wait until hot foods are cool before putting them into the refrigerator. Newer refrigerators have sufficient cooling capacity that they can handle warm foods with no problem. Don't let the temperature of your food drop below 60 °C on the countertop. Put it in the fridge right away. Refrigerated foods should be stored in small, shallow containers no deeper than 5 centimetres. Larger containers can hold heat at the centre for longer.
- Many people don't realise that leftover gravies, marinades and sauces need to be reheated to a full boil to kill germs. All leftover foods should reach a temperature of 74 °C. Just quickly warming them up in the microwave is not sufficient.
- Ensure that your food preparation counter is clean and dry. It is important to make sure that any dishes, pots, containers, Tupperware, coolers, wrappers, lunch boxes and bags that are going to come into contact with the food are clean as well.
- Tightly seal raw or undercooked meats in plastic wrap to prevent juices from coming into contact with other foods. Don't ever put a plate of raw poultry in the fridge without sealing it completely. Keep meats in a separate container at the bottom of the fridge.
- If going to a barbecue, it's best to keep the raw meats in a completely separate cooler from the other foods. The coolers must always be kept

below 4 °C. The internal temperature of a cooler left in a closed car on a sunny day can increase by 1 °C every minute. Make sure the cooler is well cleaned out with soap and water before putting the food inside.

- The safest foods to take along on a trip are shelf-stable foods such as single-serve cereals or trail mix, canned goods, peanut butter sandwiches and washed fresh fruit and vegetables.

- Never reuse the grocery bag, but dispose of it at once as it can carry the viruses of the products it contained.

- If you go to a farmers' market, go early to avoid produce that has been sitting out all day long and touched by who knows how many hands.

- Some old-world recipes such as Sauerbraten call for foods to be marinated at room temperature, some for as long as several days. Disregard that. Always marinade in the fridge.

- Hot dogs from traditional stands may taste great but many have been cooked in water that has never come to the boil, and thus are very dangerous.

- Rare hamburgers: consider them cyanide on a bun.

- Obey the expiration dates on the packaging, especially for raw poultry and meats.

- One-third of all people admit to eating pizza the next day that has spent the night at room temperature. If pizza has been out for more than two hours, it must be disposed of.

- Beware of using the microwave to defrost without thoroughly cleaning the platter and the internal surfaces before placing fresh food inside it.

- Many people think that if food is picked up from the floor within seconds, it is safe to eat. It never is.
- When dining at a buffet, remember that food should never be left out at room temperature for more than two hours. If the weather is warmer the safe time becomes shorter. It's only an hour at 32 °C.
- Double dipping, or dipping a vegetable or chip into a bowl of salsa or dip, biting some off and then dipping again, is a sure way of transmitting germs.
- Make sure your turkey stuffing reaches 74 °C all the way through. The stuffing absorbs juices from the poultry or meat and can harbour germs if not thoroughly cooked through. It's best to cook the stuffing separately and then add some hot pan drippings to moisten and flavour.
- One-quarter of all working people keep their packed lunch at their desks instead of in the fridge. Those five or six hours at room temperature is plenty of time for germs to multiply.
- The average workplace fridge is cleaned only about once in two months. All leftovers should be tossed within a few days. And beware of what is in that fridge; I knew a lab worker who kept her lunch in the refrigerator with the stool samples.
- With many markets and delis placing little nibbles of food out for tasting, most people don't realise that those samples have come into contact with countless other customers. Avoid these at all costs.
- Always place meat at the bottom of the shopping cart, or better yet, in a completely separate area.

Shop for meat, poultry and seafood just before checking out and ensure that the packaging is fully sealed and cold to the touch. Keep all meats, poultry and seafood in separate grocery bags from other foods.

- Packaged chicken should be pink, not grey or yellow. Fish should be shiny and firm and not falling from the bones. The flesh should be light pink not grey, greenish or brown. Fresh fish should not have an overly 'fishy' smell. Fish should be cooked until it is opaque and flakes easily. Never buy anything if cooked and raw produce are displayed in the same case. That applies to cooked or smoked seafood next to raw fish, or deli meats in the case with raw meat.

- There is one rule for sushi, sashimis, raw shellfish and tartares. Don't eat them!

- Some dried or cured meats can harbour countless germs. It may be a good idea to microwave these meats, then allow them to cool and consume immediately.

- Broasted chicken, ribs, etc should always be reheated to 74 °C once you are ready to eat them. Avoid purchasing whole poultry that's pre-stuffed but not cooked. The raw meat juices mixing with the stuffing, present a perfect environment for the spread of germs.

- Never eat any poultry unless all juices are running clear and not bloody at all. Rare poultry of any kind is an express ticket to the hospital.

- Store-packaged products should never be consumed raw, but must be cooked thoroughly at temperatures exceeding 77 °C.

- The average apple comes into contact with more than 50 people before you take it home and it can pick up viruses at every step of the way. All fruits and vegetables should be thoroughly washed, if possible in a light detergent dilution, not just before eating but also immediately upon arriving at home. Although fresh produce is tasty and full of natural enzymes, during a flu pandemic it is wise to avoid salads and crudités, cook or blanche all vegetables and turn all fruits into cooked compotes. Raw sprouts such as alfalfa or radish are safest when cooked.

- One-quarter of all fruit-containing cocktails and punches have not had the fruit washed. All fruit should be carefully and thoroughly washed before placing into drinks. Even if the fruit is to be peeled, it is important to wash it first to help eliminate germs that can spread through cutting and peeling. It is important to ensure that the water you are washing the fruit with is germ-free, thus sterilising tablets or other water treatment should be considered.

- Ensure that all dairy products and juices are pasteurised. Raw juices can harbour large numbers of germs. If juicing your own vegetables or fruits, wash carefully first.

- Scrub firm produce such as melons and cucumbers with a clean produce brush.

- Don't purchase any food with mould, bruises or cuts. That is an excellent breeding ground for germs.

- Remove and discard the outer leaves of lettuce.

- Keep your foods fresh. Don't stock up at bulk

stores. It's not a good idea to keep most fresh food for more than three days.

- Two-thirds of all people never wash the exteriors of cans and bottles before opening them, leaving the contents to be contaminated.
- At least once every two weeks, scrub the interior of the refrigerator including all shelves and drawers using a clean sponge and warm soapy water. A few drops of bleach in the solution will help. Rinse with plenty of clean water then dry with paper towels or a clean cloth. Make sure you carefully wipe around the corners and the fridge seals, as they can get very mouldy.
- One of the most basic food safety rules is to separate different cutting boards, dishes and utensils. This is done to minimise cross-contamination. Cross-contamination can occur if you are cutting up some raw chicken and then use the same cutting board to cut the strawberries for dessert. The germs that were present on the chicken have now contaminated the strawberries. Although the contaminants in the chicken will be killed if the chicken is cooked to 82 °C, the strawberries will be eaten raw and thus provide a direct conduit for potentially deadly germs into your system. Therefore, the best thing to do is to set up separate cutting boards, possibly colour-coded, for foods to be consumed raw and others that will be well cooked. Do the same with knives, containers and anything else that comes into contact with potentially contaminated foods. There's no point using a separate cutting board but the same knife!

- Discard old cutting boards that have cracks, crevices and excessive knife scars. Those areas can serve as a breeding ground for countless germs.
- Wash cutting boards thoroughly in hot soapy water after each use or place in dishwasher at the hottest setting available. Use a bleach solution (ie one tablespoon thin bleach in one litre of water) or other sanitising solution and rinse with clean water.
- Get a good thermometer and use it whenever you're cooking anything. Here is a guide to minimum temperatures and states of safe cooking.

Egg sauces, custards	71 °C
Beef, veal, lamb and pork	71 °C
Ham – fresh (raw)	71 °C
Ham – fully cooked (to reheat)	60 °C
Chicken, turkey, duck and goose	82 °C
Stuffing – cooked alone or in bird	74 °C
Sauces, soups, gravies and marinades	Bring to a boil
Fin fish	Cook until opaque and flakes easily with a fork
Shrimp, lobster and crab	Should turn red and flesh should become pearly opaque
Scallops	Should turn milky white or opaque and firm
Clams, mussels and oysters	Cook until shells open
Leftovers	74 °C

Eggs: Tasty, convenient, nutritious virus reservoirs

Eggs definitely merit their own section. Fully cooked eggs cannot contain active virus. The problem is that infective viruses can be transmitted by insufficiently cooked eggs and improper handling during preparation.

One of the great joys of my life has been devouring chocolate chip cookie dough. I could never get enough. The same went for licking out the cake batter bowl. For one birthday, my wife made me a lemon cake but didn't bake it. She just handed me the bowl with a spoon. Happy Birthday! But also Happy Contamination. I now realise that these raw foods contain equally raw eggs, which are extremely dangerous and should never be eaten unless fully cooked.

Here is the cardinal rule of eggs: never ever eat raw eggs or anything that has raw eggs in it, including cookie dough and homemade cookie dough ice cream. Don't follow Rocky Balboa's example by downing a glass of raw eggs to build up your muscles. All you are doing is building up your viral titre (level within your body).

When you're selecting eggs at the market always choose a carton that is cold to the touch and make sure the eggs are clean and aren't broken or cracked. Chicken faeces on the eggshell the size of the nail on your little finger can contain millions of live H5N1 viruses.

If a recipe calls for raw eggs, for example Caesar salad dressing or a zabaglione, you can use liquid pasteurised egg substitute instead.

When you get home, place the eggs in the coldest part of the refrigerator in their original packaging, not in the moulded-in eggcups in the door, which can stay several degrees warmer. Furthermore, the fridge eggcups can transfer contaminants from one set of eggs to the next.

Raw eggs should not be kept for more than three weeks in the refrigerator, however, hard-boiled eggs can last a week. Just to be on the safer side, I'd cut these times in half.

When you're cooking eggs, whether fried, poached or whatever, make sure that you continue cooking them until the yolks are firm. If you like runny yolks, then re-learn to like them hard – or switch your breakfast to cereal instead. When you're preparing egg dishes like quiches, ensure that they reach a minimum of 71 °C all the way through.

Since H5N1 is originally an avian virus, the recent penchant for free-range eggs sourced directly from small farms presents a significant infection potential. Unlike large-scale commercial eggs that are usually mechanically washed, these eggs are often soiled with significant amounts of bird faeces, which can contain lethal amounts of H5N1. Contact with H5N1 infected poultry faeces was recently found to be the source of infection and death among victims in Asia. Handling the eggs with rubber gloves is not enough as the contents of the egg wrap themselves around the edge of the shell through surface tension when the egg is cracked, transporting live virus directly into your recipe. Eggs should be thoroughly scrubbed with hot water and soap before use. If you find that the hot water partially cooks the egg and ruins the recipe, then it might be time to change your recipe.

Most of the world's governments will try to do everything possible to prevent the spread of avian flu and we can count on many of the major supermarket chains to offer eggs for sale that have been subjected to the same proper hygienic conditions that protect from salmonella and campylobacter, which will also protect from avian flu. The problem may be concentrated on eggs sourced from small, family farms and similar free-range chicken operations. On the main road near my home in Dorset, England, there is a small farm selling fresh eggs that are literally caked in faeces.

Remember: Runny poached eggs or fried eggs, French toast, Caesar salad and zabagliones using raw or barely cooked eggs would be a direct conduit for H5N1 into your system. Avoid them like the plague or the plague won't avoid you!

CHAPTER 7

When Home Treatment is the Only Option

Providing basic health care to your family once the medical system is swamped

To qualify as a new pandemic three criteria must be met:

- The infectious agent must be a new virus that the majority of the population is susceptible to and one for which there is no effective vaccine.
- The virus must be able to replicate in humans and cause disease.
- The virus must be easily transmitted from person to person.

Once you are made aware through the news media that the last phase has occurred, you must then prepare yourself for providing basic medical care to your family and loved ones who may become infected with H5N1. By that time the medical system of your country will be swamped. Every estimate of daily visits to the doctor during a pandemic is off the scale. Doctors will be booked solid for months and empty hospital beds will be nonexistent. There will be a very lucky few who will be able to receive quality medical care during a pandemic. The rest of us will essentially be on our own. By all means, try everything in your power to get medical attention, but keep these techniques in mind as a fallback.

There are basic techniques that you can use in your own home to help minimise the spread of H5N1 from members of your family who have become infected, as well as make them as comfortable as possible.

The first aspect you must implement is the use of barrier nursing, or bedside isolation. This is a set of techniques to protect the caregiver and the rest of the environment from infection by contagious persons. Essentially the procedures utilised in barrier nursing are rather common sense. The basic goal is to create a barrier to the transmission of germs between the contagious patient and their caregivers and the rest of their environment.

The preferred method is to isolate the patient in their own room, but when that becomes impossible and several patients must be present in a ward, then the best practice is to place screens around each bed.

The caregivers have to follow strict regulations to keep the transmission of infectious agents at a minimum. Anything that comes into contact with the patient must be sterilised, either by immediately placing any equipment or utensils touched by the patient in a bowl of disinfectant or by outright incineration. Caregivers must practise meticulous and prompt handwashing techniques. Any bedding should be carefully moved and placed directly into sealed biohazard-marked bags as vigorous bed changing can spread contaminants. Laundering of any textiles that have come into contact with the patient must be cleaned in special facilities that use steam heat or very hot water for sterilisation. If incineration is an option it should be used. Spills of blood, vomit or any other bodily fluid should be cleaned up promptly with a disinfectant solution such as 1:10 dilution of bleach. Extreme care must be used in the disposal of faeces. Remember that absolutely everything that comes into contact with the patient or issues from the patient may be highly infectious.

The caregivers must at all times that they are in the presence of the patient be outfitted with full surgical gowns, respirators, eye or face protection and rubber gloves. A makeshift surgical gown can easily be made out of a clean bed sheet.

Detailed information on respirators can be found on page 64. Goggles must fit securely and should be of the indirectly vented type. Directly vented goggles may allow splashes or sprays to enter the eye and are to be avoided. There are special types of goggles that will go over prescription glasses while maintaining a tight fit, therefore if you are a glasses wearer, they are well worth seeking out. There are also face shields that are designed for infection control. They are usually quite large and cover the entire face from crown to chin.

Eye and face protection should always be removed by handling only the strap that holds the device to the head. The fronts and sides of the item may have become contaminated with droplets during the caring for the patient and can be highly infectious. All of these items must be sterilised after each and every use according to the manufacturers' instructions.

Gloves should be put on well in advance of touching any patient when there is even the slightest risk of coming into contact with blood or any other bodily fluids. The only bodily fluid that can be considered safe is perspiration, but all others, including blood, saliva, vomit, urine or faeces must be considered a clear biohazard. It is always a good idea to wear gloves, even if there are no contaminated fluids present, as the situation can readily change when caring for an H5N1 patient. The disease profoundly affects the entire body and the patient may vomit, excrete or bleed with no warning. Keep the gloves securely on during the entire time that you are in contact with the patient and do not touch anything else while wearing the gloves. After the encounter is over the gloves that have come into contact with the patient are considered severely contaminated, therefore anything that the gloves have come into contact with or will come into contact with can also be considered contaminated. You must be meticulously aware of what you have used when you were wearing your gloves, including basic items that you usually don't give a second thought to, such as pens or paper pads. If you have a medical kit make sure that you don't contaminate it by accessing it with your gloves on.

The caregiver must pay particular attention to preventing any problems aside from contagious viruses; 1 per cent of the general population and 10 per cent of health care professionals suffer from latex allergy, the substance used in rubber gloves and over 50,000 other products. Latex sensitivity can present itself as an irritant dermatitis, which in itself is not an allergic but a skin reaction, where small breaks in the skin surface allow latex proteins into the skin. There is also the possibility of contact dermatitis, although the occurrence of this may be linked to various additives in the rubber processing rather than the latex itself. The industry is minimising the use of these additives, so this particular reaction is diminishing. The most severe reaction is immediate hypersensitivity where serious swelling, reddening and itching of the affected skin can occur. There is a raft of associated problems that sometimes manifest themselves, including asthma, rhinitis, bronchial spasms and even fatal anaphylactic shock.

The room the patient resides in must have plenty of fresh air. To assess the total air in the room, a measurement of air changes per hour (ACH – how much fresh outside air enters a room in an hour) is made. A 3.7 metre square normal room will contain over 31.1 cubic metres of air, so a single air change means that 31.1 cubic metres of fresh, clean air vented directly from the outside will enter the room each and every hour. The absolute minimum for a contagious patient room is 6 ACH (which would require 186.6 cubic metres of fresh air every hour), but 12 is preferred (373.2 cubic metres). That is an amazingly large amount of air. In the latter example that translates to replacing every single bit of air in the room every five minutes. In the wintertime when we are accustomed to hermetically sealing up all the windows, some rooms can drop to 0.25 ACH – that's only six air changes per day.

The best way to ensure this amount of fresh air is to keep a window in the patient's room at least halfway open and to shelter the patient's bed from any cold drafts by screens and additional space heating if required.

The patient must be kept comfortable, clean, well fed and hydrated. Make sure that there is always plenty of cool, fresh water available. Conventional cold and flu medications are quite useless against H5N1, but painkillers may relieve pain and discomfort. Don't overdose the patient on antihistamines, decongestants and similar drugs. You will find that they will be better off without them.

Have a comprehensive first aid kit available and well stocked. It would also be prudent to take a first-aid course in your area. Critical situations can arise swiftly and without warning.

This is a short chapter because there really isn't much more that you can do. The disease must run its course. There are precious few procedures that are carried out even in intensive care wards that go far beyond these basics. H5N1 is a frightful illness, but it must be remembered that if the mortality rate matches both expectations and the precedents of the great pandemics of the past, nine out of ten infected patients will recover. And those are pretty good odds!

CHAPTER 8

Home and Alternative Remedies

Folk remedies may not help, but can they hurt?

Kimchi is the Korean national dish and is made by fermenting cabbage in vinegar with red peppers, radishes and a lot of garlic and ginger. I first became acquainted with the dish on a stopover at Seoul Airport and now I'm incredibly fond of it, although most Westerners I know think it's horrific rubbish. However, there may now be a new reason to devour kimchi with the same gusto as Koreans.

Professor Kang Sa-ouk at Seoul National University fed an extract of kimchi to H5N1 infected chickens and a week later 90 per cent of them had started recovering. 'We found that the chickens recovered from bird flu, Newcastle disease and bronchitis. The birds' death rate fell, they were livelier and their stools became normal,' he said. There was a marked increase in kimchi consumption when thousands of people in Asia contracted SARS (Severe Acute Respiratory Syndrome). Now, thanks to Professor Kang's study, South Koreans are reported to be eating even more kimchi and maybe even feeding it to their backyard poultry.

There are countless home and folk remedies that are as controversial as the kimchi cure. Each remedy has its supporters and some may even claim to have scientific clinical proof of their efficacy. No respectable practitioner should ever claim that they can cure a case of H5N1 infection, as that has been proven to be impossible by any measurement of modern science. These various folk and alternative medical products may alleviate symptoms in some cases and do absolutely nothing in other cases. The bottom line is *caveat emptor*: let the buyer beware. There is no conclusive evidence in current medical literature that any of these remedies do anything but leave your wallet thinner. Some of them may actually pose an element of danger; some Indian Ayurvedic medicines have recently been found to contain unacceptably high concentrations of heavy metals. However, you will find thousands, if not millions, of people that swear by each of these remedies and, in the case of most of them, they may have no beneficial effect but they probably can't hurt. If you think that they will make you feel better then they may be worth investigating for your own personal use.

Therefore, for the rest of this chapter, we will be discarding scientific caution. These remedies and the claims made for them are listed for educational use and specifically not indicated to cure anything. I'm not going to use 'alleged' and other similar terms, otherwise each sentence may have multiple 'alleged's in it. So remember that these are based on folklore, rather than scientific fact and each remedy should be considered as 'alleged'.

Homeopathy

Homeopathy was founded in the early 19th century by a German physician, Dr Hahnemann. It swiftly became so popular that in the late 19th century 15 per cent of the doctors in the US were homeopaths. A recent study published in August 2005 in the prestigious medical journal *The Lancet* showed that homeopathic remedies and placebos have no significant difference in efficacy, but that is not expected to put a dent into the popularity of this alternative medicine.

Classical homeopathy is based on three basic principles: the law of similars, the single medicine, and the minimum dose.

The law of similars states that a disease is best cured by a substance that causes symptoms similar to that disease in a normally healthy person. That is the basis for the lengthy interviews that homeopaths give their patients in order to determine the exact symptoms that they are presenting with. Once all the information is gathered, the homeopath determines which remedy best matches the symptoms the patient has described.

The principle of the single remedy basically states that a single medicine must address all the symptoms the patient is experiencing: mental, emotional, and physical. In classical homeopathy two remedies would not be prescribed for two different symptoms. The homeopath would prescribe a single medicine that covered both symptoms.

The principle of the minimum dose is twofold: to begin with, the homeopath prescribes a small number of doses of the remedy and measures the effect it has. If the homeopath derives the desired result, the remedy is prescribed in an infinitesimal dose. Apparently, the effect of homeopathic remedies is strengthened upon successive dilutions as long as the compound is subject to strong shaking between each dilution. Remedies are typically used in very high dilutions such as 200C, which means that the original substance has been diluted in water at a 100 to 1 concentration for 200 consecutive times. That makes a dilution of 10 to the 400th power. To put this into perspective: there are 10 to the 70th power atoms in the entire galaxy. So this is a concentration of far, far less than a single atom in the entire Milky Way.

This infinitesimal dosing is the most controversial aspect of homeopathy. There have been determinations that in samples of remedies at 200C virtually not a single molecule of the original substance is present. However, there are millions of people all over the world who insist that homeopathic remedies are very effective due to the 'memory' aspect of water that 'remembers' what was in it, and they disregard the chemists who state that they are ingesting nothing but pure water.

There are many homeopathic flu remedies, but Oscillococcinum (also called Anas barbariae) is generally regarded to be the Gold Standard. In Continental Europe, especially France, it is widely believed to decrease the duration and intensity of flu symptoms. Oscillococcinum has quickly become the number one flu medicine in France, outselling any other natural or conventional medicine, and on this strength is becoming increasingly popular around the world. Oscillococcinum is an extract of Barbary duck heart and liver diluted 200 times at 100 to one (200C). It was introduced in the 1930s by Dr Joseph Roy, who believed that it contained the bacterium Oscillococcus, which at that time was thought to cause influenza. The connection between the avian source of this remedy and the common carrier of H5N1 definitely gives cause to reflect.

Herbal remedies

Herbal medicine is also known as Botanical or Phytomedicine. It refers to a part of a plant that can be used essentially unprocessed to promote the healing from a particular ailment. The basis of about a quarter of all common pharmaceuticals is herbal and usually comes from a tropical environment such as the Amazonian rainforest. Three-quarters of these drugs were developed by investigating medical folklore claims.

Phytomedicine is the oldest form of healthcare known to mankind. Herbs had been used by all cultures throughout history to alleviate disease. It was an integral part of the development of modern civilisation. Four out of five people on Earth still rely on herbal sources as their primary medicine.

Much of the medicinal use of plants seems to have been developed through the centuries via observations of the behaviour of wild animals, and by trial and error. Each human tribe added the medicinal power of herbs in their area to its repertory, transmitted first orally, then in written form, which methodically collected information on herbs to develop extensive and accurate profiles of each. Well into the 20th century much of the medical pharmacopoeia was a direct extrapolation from herbal native folklore.

In 1874 the German Egyptologist Georg Ebers discovered a 65-foot papyrus, which was dated to approximately 1,500 BC. The Ebers Papyrus contains information of a millennium of medical history and practice in Egypt and describes 876 herbal formulations made from more than 500 plants. Almost half of these herbs are listed in today's Western pharmacopoeia.

Modern herbal medicines are standardised to a great degree, ensuring consistent potency and safety. There are millions of people who turn to these compounds for relief from the symptoms of flu. The most popular of these may be Echinacea (*Echinacea purpurea*) especially when taken in conjunction with Goldenseal (*Hydrastis canadensis*).

Traditional Chinese medicine

The origins of Chinese herbalism are unknown to historians, but according to legend the mythological Emperor Shen Nung invented agriculture in approximately 3500 BC, and had begun to explore the medicinal properties of different plants. He authored China's first great herbal text, the *Pen Tsao Ching* (The Classic of Herbs). This publication described 237 herbal prescriptions composed from scores of herbs. Each subsequent emperor continued with this tradition, and by 1590 AD, Li Shin-Chen published a 52-volume *Pen Tsao Kang Mu* (The Catalogue of Medicinal Herbs), containing 1,094 medicinal plants and more than 11,000 diverse medicinal formulas.

The Traditional Chinese Medicine (TCM) approach varies significantly to the very concept of Western medicine. TCM views the human body as a single, integrated organism and within it each organ is a complex structure, which manifests itself not only physiologically and functionally, but also through emotion, colour, climate and milieu.

TCM and Western medicine developed along very different lines. While Western doctors were learning about the body through dissection and analysis, surgical interventions were discouraged in TCM, focusing on symptoms not the underlying organs.

Some of the traditional compounds used in TCM to fight the flu include:

- Gan Mao Ling: This is one of the most popular and trusted Chinese patents for chills and high fever, fatigue, swollen lymph glands, sore throats and back and neck aches. If taken prior to the onset of the flu it is believed to prevent these symptoms.

- Yin Chiao: In a similar manner to Gan Mao Ling, Yin Chiao is regularly prescribed in the flu symptoms of headaches, sore throats, body aches, fever with chills, unreasonable thirst, stiff neck and shoulders. Yin Chiao is best taken at the first signs of flu symptoms.

Ayurvedic medicine

In Ancient India, starting 50 centuries ago, medicine was called Ayurveda. In Sanskrit *ayur* means 'life' and *veda* stands for 'knowledge', thus Ayurveda is the 'science of life'. Ayurvedic medicine was based on four Vedas, which were books of classic wisdom. The first of these volumes, the *Rig Veda*, includes detailed descriptions of procedures such as amputation, eye surgeries, and other operations that would be right at home in a modern hospital.

The *Rig Veda* also contains descriptions of 67 different herbs such as ginger, cinnamon and senna. From this long-standing history, Ayurveda today is still based on the principle of eternal life through a symbiosis of mind, body and spirit. Ayurvedic practitioners believe that any imbalance in this synthesis results in physical diseases.

There are three founding texts for Ayurvedic medicine. *Charaka Samhita* was written in its latest form approximately 2,000 years ago, and was followed by the *Vagbhatta's Astanga Hridaya* five centuries later and the *Susruta Samhita* two centuries after that. These texts are believed to have originated from many centuries before these dates, but were rewritten and revised up to these dates. These three classic texts contain extensive clinical as well as surgical information on an encyclopaedic collection of diseases and ailments.

Ayurvedic medicine seeks to establish and maintain a balance of humours and detoxification of the body, thus features preventative as well as curative measures.

Some Ayurvedic medicinal compounds have been recently accused of containing elevated levels of dangerous heavy metals, thus they are not currently recommended. Regardless, the compounds that are indicated for the prevention and alleviation of flu symptoms are many and include Sitopaladi Churna, a preparation with readily available ingredients such as cardamom, cinnamon and raw brown sugar. Sitopaladi Churna is unusual among Ayurvedic compounds in that it is absolutely delicious with a sweet spiciness, unlike the bitter quality of most of these types of medicines. The average dose is a teaspoon of the powder two to four times daily, but you may find yourself eating more, as it's almost a candy. It might not do a thing against H5N1 but at least it's tasty.

There are two other ingredients, which are not common in Western markets but are easily found in most Indian or Chinese ethnic shops: bamboo manna (*Phyllostachys Nigra*), which is the inner sap of bamboo (called Zhu Li in TCM), and pippli pepper (*Piper Longum*, called Bi Ba in TCM), which is a perennial climbing plant with fleshy fruits.

Remedies that cross boundaries

Some herbs are shared by both Ayurveda and TCM. The most popular against flu are:

- Astragalus (*Astragalus membranaceus* or Huang Qi in TCM), which is prescribed mainly for long-term disease prevention and for acute flu symptoms. Astragalus enhances immune function by facilitating the activity of some white blood cells, which in turn increases the production of antibodies, and it also increases the production of interferon (an antiviral substance naturally produced by the body).

- Andrographis (*Andrographis paniculata*), which is a very widely used medicine in both Ayurveda and TCM, and has been a household remedy in Asia for many centuries. In Ayurveda, which calls it 'kalmegh' (king of the bitters), it is used for upper respiratory infection (flu, bronchitis). TCM utilises Andrographis for fever and headache from colds and flu, tonsillitis, laryngopharyngitis, bronchitis and inflammation.

This has served only a brief overview of some of the alternative medicine therapies claimed to be successful in beating the flu. Some of the other disciplines include:

Acupressure
Aromatherapy
Bach flower remedies
Essential oils
Hydrotherapy
Imagery
Juice therapy
Naturopathy
Reflexology
Sound therapy
Tissue Salts
Yoga

Then there are some that really don't fit into any of the categories above.

Propolis

Propolis is a blend of resinous sap from trees, beeswax, and enzymes produced by the bees. Propolis has antiviral, antibacterial and antifungal properties. The bees use propolis to protect their hive residents from infections. Beehives are one of the most sterile environments known, and this is largely attributed to the antibiotic properties of propolis. It is usually taken for antibiotic purposes in tablet form, as a tincture to apply to wounds and rashes, or as a supplement to skin lotions, shampoos, toothpaste, etc.

Zinc

Zinc appears to have particular salubrious effects on the immune system and it may have a direct virucidal effect. Zinc preparations in lozenge or nasal gel form are now available as flu treatments. Zinc should not be taken for reasons other than flu or for any longer than is strictly necessary.

Vitamin C

I once had the pleasure of meeting Dr Linus Pauling, the Nobel Prize-winning author of the bestselling *Vitamin C, The Common Cold and the Flu*, where he advocates extremely high doses of Vitamin C to ward off and cure flu. Some recent research has shown that high vitamin doses may be dangerous.

Wacky pseudo-remedies from generations of sheer quacks

Then of course there are those who come up with the most unlikely and ridiculous, if not outright dangerous, pseudo-remedies. I cannot possibly stress enough how any of these may be unsafe in a variety of ways and there is not one shred of clinical evidence to show that they do anything beneficial at all. I do not recommend that you even consider trying any of these for any reason at any time. Please note that if you try any of these pseudo-remedies, you do so at your physiological and psychological peril!

Hydrogen Peroxide In Your Ear

In 1928, a Dr Richard Simmons hypothesised that flu virus enters the human body through the ear canal and not through the eyes, nose or mouth as convention-al knowledge dictates. Dr Simmons' findings were dismissed by the medical community. According to Dr Simmons, keeping your fingers out of your ears will greatly reduce your chances of catching the flu. Once the viruses have entered the inner ear, they then begin to multiply and have access to the rest of the body from there.

Remarkable results are claimed to be achieved in cur-ing the flu outright within 12 hours by administering a few drops of 3 per cent Hydrogen Peroxide (H_2O_2) into each ear. There will be some bubbling and in some cases mild stinging might occur. Then you wait until the bub-bling subsides in a few minutes, then drain onto a tissue and repeat with the other ear.

Cod Liver Oil

Two tablespoons of this infamous old-school remedy into a glass of orange juice with a splash of wine vinegar. Take every 12 hours.

Colloidal Silver

Basically the same compound that is used in hot tub and spa sanitation, taken internally or even injected.

Cannabis

Smoking cannabis or marijuana is believed to keep you free from flu.

Orgone Electronic

A Mobius coil triggers a crystal through a magnet that releases the energy of Orgone to cure you.

1918 Flu Pandemic Folk Cures (Emphatically not recommended!)

- Gargle with bicarbonate of soda, boric acid and chlorinated soda.
- Eat sugar laced with turpentine or kerosene.
- Eat copious amounts of porridge.
- Inhale tobacco smoke.
- Spray either a mixture of carbolic acid and quinine or sodium bicarbonate mixed with boric acid in your nose.
- Wear necklaces adorned with sacks of garlic, goose grease or camphor balls.
- Burn and inhale sulphur or brown sugar.
- Sleep over a shotgun so the steel of the gun will draw out the fever.
- Sweat continuously for 90 minutes.
- Stand outside in the cold, naked.
- Drink a solution of citrate of potash.
- Inhale vapours from a pepper stew.
- Drink lots of alcohol.

- Eat compressed yeast.
- Lie in a tub full of chopped onions.

You can have a look on any major internet search engine for cures that are guaranteed to cure the flu. At a recent count there were 32,581 websites that supposedly offered immunity or outright cure from H5N1 (for a small, nominal charge on your Visa, Mastercard or Paypal account).

Of course we can't forget the world's favourite healing soup: chicken soup. It has often been called Yiddish penicillin for its miraculous soothing medicinal qualities, and, after centuries of folklore, medical science has finally proven that chicken soup combats the symptoms of a cold. Dr Stephen Rennard, an American pulmonary specialist, tested various chicken soups in the laboratory. He found that the soups had anti-inflammatory properties, helping to soothe sore throats and stop the movement of neutrophils, the white blood cells that encourage the flow of mucus that accumulates in the lungs and nose.

Listings on where to obtain the products discussed in this section can be found in the Resources.

CHAPTER 9

The Only Effective Antivirals?

How to get the only drugs that might help while scant stocks still exist

Roche's Tamiflu (*oseltamivir phosphate*) is one of only two pharmaceuticals known to have a measure of efficacy against the majority of H5N1 variants. As a neuraminidase inhibitor, it works by binding to the N mushrooms on the surface of the virus particles, almost as if it were clogging them. By interfering in this way with the N mushrooms on the surface, which are used by H5N1 to leave the infected cell, they can't go on to infect more. If the baby viruses can't break out of the tough living cell membrane they get stuck in there and can't get out.

Tamiflu is best used when symptoms of flu first appear, but it is also useful in reducing the chances of contracting H5N1 during a pandemic. Therefore it fits two separate profiles. The first is the conventional drug. You have symptoms, you take the pill, and you might get better. The second is what is known as a prophylaxis, which is the drug that you take when you are perfectly healthy in order to keep you from getting the disease. This twofold effect is what makes neuraminidase inhibitors the most powerful agent in the fight against H5N1 and therefore so sought after.

The Only Effective Antivirals?

Neuraminidase inhibitors confine the infection to a smaller area of your body, making the symptoms of the infection less severe, as the effects of the drug make it easier for your immune system to finish the virus off. Studies have demonstrated that the drug reduces the length of the flu by approximately one day, and reduces the risk of developing complications such as chest infections that require antibiotics.

It is important to note that the dosage must be rather elevated. Studies have shown that the commonly prescribed dosage still means that 50 per cent of the subjects tested against virulent strains of H5N1 will die. The currently recommended dosage is one 75-milligram pill per day for a month minimum as soon as the pandemic hits your geographical area (as a prophylaxis) and four pills per day for a week as soon as you start to show symptoms. Since the price of the drug averages £4/$7.20 per pill, this can soon add up. At the time of this book going to press, a clinical report has been issued stating that this dose is too low and should be increased many-fold. However, let's continue these calculations on the smaller, previously recommended dosage.

If the pandemic hits your area two months before you contract it, and you have symptoms for ten days (which is the 'expected case'), the cost could be over £400/$720. In our affluent society, it's a small price to pay in order to derive the benefits, but in parts of the Third World that is over a year's salary. In some 'worse case' scenarios, the pandemic lasts six months and the flu symptoms can stretch to almost a month, which would call for almost £900 /$1,620 of the drug per person.

However, both the affluent and developing countries will have a problem greater than affording the drug. To be fair to Roche, they just contributed 30 million Tamiflu pills to the WHO, but they won't actually be able to produce that much drug for several years. To date, the WHO has only received enough to treat 125,000 people with the minimum dosage possible of ten pills each.

Roche's Chief Executive Officer William M Burns stated in July 2005: 'We've never actually released what our capacity is, nor do we intend to. The question we ask governments is, "What do you want?" And if you give us orders, we will ensure that we put in place the supply chain to meet that.' The single Swiss Roche plant that manufactures Tamiflu is at 100 per cent capacity. The current production rate for Tamiflu before the increases that Roche is 'planning' has been 'rumoured' to be 1.5 million doses per year. Note that is not 1.5 million people's full courses, but individual doses. Given the fact that the most basic legitimate number of doses for two months of prophylaxis and a very short ten days of symptoms is 100 pills, this only covers 15,000 people.

In October 2005 Roche announced that they were willing to license the manufacture of Tamiflu to other pharmaceutical companies – Barr, Teva, Mylan, Ranbaxy and others. This news was widely lauded, but in the words of John Milligan, chief financial officer of Gilead Sciences Inc, whose company developed Tamiflu, 'I don't think it's the quick fix that countries are looking for.' According to Terence Hurley, a spokesman for Roche, getting new facilities approved to produce Tamiflu can take up to 15 months and, once approved, new batches will take as long as a year to produce, since manufacturing Tamiflu involves controlled chemical explosions, at least five different production sites, seven manufacturers besides Roche itself and raw materials from 40 suppliers. Therefore, the earliest that Tamiflu could be produced by licensees is over two years away, and the amount produced will only be incremental, not the many orders of magnitude required. Taiwan was the first government to announce that they were going to go ahead with Tamiflu production without any license from Roche, a move that violates international patent law. At about the same time, Roche announced that they had stopped shipping Tamiflu to most of their biggest customers, allegedly to stop private hoarding in order to preserve numbers for government shipments. More than a few analysts saw the Roche move as a way to put pressure on any potential patent infringers, such as Taiwan, since it would be a long time until any Tamiflu-clone facility (coined 'Taiflu' by some observers) could come onstream.

The World Population Clock as I write this stands at 6,548,556,472. That means that there is enough Tamiflu currently being produced per year to treat only one out of over 436,570 people. To put that into perspective there is only enough Tamiflu produced a year worldwide to treat just one person in every city the size of Oslo.

If Roche were to announce that it is ramping up its production by an unprecedented 1,000-fold (next to impossible in practical production terms within even a five-year span) all that would mean is that 1,000 people in Oslo would get the basic dose and 435,570 still would not. Let's project the completely impossibly mad prospect that Roche could increase its production 100,000-fold. You still have 336,570 people in Oslo without the basic doses of Tamiflu.

Unfortunately, Roche's licensee program is likely to only increase the manufacturing capacity of Tamiflu 20-fold at best, and that in two years. Good news for 20 people in

Oslo, but bad news for the other 436,550. Even possible clone factories are unlikely to be able to do much better than that.

US President Bush announced in November 2005 that he would ask Congress for an additional $7.1 billion over and above the billions the US Senate had already approved for emergency flu measure. At least $3.9 billion is earmarked for the stockpiling of antivirals, a stunning sum that was certain to be greeted with glee in pharmaceutical boardrooms. Yet even that amount, if used to purchase Tamiflu at market price and if there were that much Tamiflu in existence, would only result in less than three pills per American. If used for prophylaxis, would be sufficient for less than 1 out of 100 people in the US. The situation is pretty much the same in other developed countries. If used for full prophylaxis, France has ordered enough for 1 out of 249 citizens, Japan 1 out of 176, Canada 1 out of 142, the UK 1 out of 61 and the Netherlands 1 out of 45.

The situation elsewhere on Earth is much worse. Indonesia, which has already suffered human H5N1 deaths, has 10,000 Tamiflu tablets, enough for 71 citizens out of its 244 million or about 1 person out of 3.5 million. The WHO's physical stockpile is currently only 800,000 pills or full prophylaxis for 5,700 individuals amidst the 6.5 billion on Earth. The majority of the world's 193 nations, specifically in South America, Africa and South Asia, have no Tamiflu at all.

I'm certain that some people will be arguing with my calculations, showing that the Tamiflu available and in the process of being manufactured by Roche, along with its new international partners and the patent-violating clone factories, will be sufficient for expected needs. To those people, I'll give you the following set of figures to cogitate. Based on 100 75-milligram pills per person to allow for a more reasonable three months of prophylaxis and ten days of four pills per day in reserve if and when they start showing symptoms, Roche should license and produce 917,797,906,080 pills (almost 917 billion pills), which works out to just about 70 million kilograms of pills or the equivalent to the total weight of the QE2 cruise ship fully loaded with passengers and cargo – in nothing other than Tamiflu pills. This is a very difficult, if not outright impossible, ramp up from their current production for Roche or any other pharmaceutical company. Not even to mention that the legitimate production and distribution cost of a single pill of Tamiflu is approximately £1.00/$1.80, which means that this much Tamiflu would cost over £915 billion/$1.65 trillion to produce.

A word of warning to those who believe that all we need is a single 'course' per person of Tamiflu and all will be well. The course of this type of influenza is typically a couple of weeks. Tamiflu can shorten that by a little over a day. That's it. It doesn't stop the influenza, it only cuts the duration of symptoms by about 10 per cent. The best use is as a prophylaxis where it must be taken daily throughout the period of time that H5N1 is present in your geographical area. I'm using two or three months as an estimate but that time could easily be doubled or tripled as no one knows how many waves this pandemic will arrive in, or how long each wave will last. Every additional month is an extra 30 pills per person. At these doses, the mortality rate is still 50 per cent against a control group. Somewhat better results can be seen at doses higher than that, prescribed by the US Food and Drug Association, but then you're faced with the prospect of doubling or tripling the amount of drug needed per individual. If we use a double-dose calculation in a six-month pandemic period and a two-week flu duration we have two pills per day for 180 days and then eight pills per day for 14 days, which adds up to 472 pills per person. We've already acknowledged that at the currently prescribed low doses, the 'cruise ship' amount is an unreachable production target, so when we get to two, three, four or more 'cruise ships' it simply abandons the realms of reality.

No matter how the numbers get switched around, the fact that the overwhelming majority of the population of the Earth will never get to see a single tablet of Tamiflu is indisputable. It just can't be done! Certainly not in this decade. In fact, the WHO estimates that it will take ten years to produce 13 billion tablets of Tamiflu. That would provide just ten pills to 20 per cent of the world's population, or prophylaxis as above to only 1.5 per cent of the people on the planet. And in the intervening decade, the pandemic may have come and gone.

However, even for the people lucky enough to get their doses, Tamiflu is far from perfect. It may cause mild to moderate nausea or vomiting in one out of ten people and could also cause rashes, abdominal pain, bronchitis, sleeplessness and vertigo. It's a good idea to take this drug with meals, as it helps to abate the side effects. It's also not recommended for pregnant or lactating women. It's also not been proven if it's safe or even if it works as a prophylaxis on children or if it works at all in babies.

If that wasn't bad enough, William Chui, honorary associate professor with the department of pharmacology at the Queen Mary Hospital in Hong Kong, says: 'There are now resistant H5N1 strains appearing, and we can't totally rely on one drug (Tamiflu).' Thus all of this may be moot as the strain of H5N1 that finally becomes pandemic may be resistant to the best drugs we have in our arsenal.

So Tamiflu can cause rather unpleasant side effects while it shortens the duration of flu symptoms by just one day and still lets half the people treated die, and that's only if the virus doesn't become resistant to it before it hits. Still, it's a little bit better than nothing and it's the best we have.

Relenza (*zanamivir*) is currently vying for the number one position with Tamiflu as the antiviral of choice against H5N1. This drug was largely disregarded until a recent study published in the medical journal *The Lancet* demonstrated virtually equal efficacy to Tamiflu in inhibiting the N mushrooms in an effectively identical manner. The developer of the drug, Biota in Australia, was actually suing the distributor, giant GlaxoSmithKline, for inadequately promoting the drug at first, selling under £2/$3.6 million worth of it worldwide, which in the mega-billion-dollar world of pharmaceuticals is like opening your hot dog stand at the stadium and selling two a day. *The Lancet* study may make the Australians happier since within days of its publication the German government ordered almost 2 million doses and many others are expected to follow suit.

Relenza is quite similar in action against H5N1 to Tamiflu but it is not a pill. It comes in a strange, disc-shaped inhaler. The process to self-administer Relenza is more than a bit puzzling. First you have to pull off the disc's blue half-moon shaped cover and check that the inhaler is not blocked. Then you extend the mouthpiece by pulling on a white tray. Then you have to locate tiny ridges on the sides of the inhaler, press them both at the same time and pull the whole thing apart. Then you have to take a silver disc that contains the actual medicine and place it right-side up atop a rotating plastic thing that looks like a flattened version of an old super-8mm movie reel and align it with the holes underneath. Then you push the whole assembly back together. You have to keep the dispenser level or the drug will spill out. You have to lift another half-circle flap and lift it up from the outer edge until it sticks straight up. Then you push it back down again. While keeping the dispenser level you have to put the mouthpiece into your mouth without covering the small holes on the sides and inhale and hold it in your lungs for a while. Then you exhale. But you're not done yet. The usual dose is two inhalations, so you have to do it all over again, including reloading the drug. You pull the mouthpiece to extend the tray again, then push it back in to rotate the disc and go inhale it some more. In most cases you need to do two more inhalations just two hours later. Before you use it the next time you have to check to see if all four blisters on the drug disc have been broken, in which case you have to start the whole process again to load a new dose of medicine.

I can certainly understand the pharmaceutical reasons why the compound within Relenza wouldn't work as a pill like Tamiflu, but there are many different ways of designing a drug inhaler and Relenza's is the most complex one I have ever seen. Although Glaxo can probably produce a stack of internal studies to prove that the inhaler is used correctly by the patients who are prescribed it, I have yet to meet a single person I have shown the Relenza inhaler to that can figure out how to use it. I can certainly understand why Glaxo was unable to sell these things before *The Lancet* study. Relenza's chemical composition does require the rupturing of a blister immediately prior to inhalation so conventional asthma-type simple inhalers wouldn't work. However, a simple design revamp to something more akin to a familiar asthma inhaler would make Relenza far more user-friendly, thus have a greater degree of successful self-administration.

Glaxo's Vice-President, Dr Allen Roses, publicly stated in 2003 that for 'the vast majority of drugs, more than 90 per cent, only work in 30 or 50 per cent of the people'. This is hardly reassuring, regardless of Glaxo's stated ability to produce more Relenza than Roche can provide Tamiflu.

Another factor to consider is that both Relenza and Tamiflu have a common problem that could severely impair the efficiency of both drugs. They start to break down if they're exposed to temperatures below 15 °C or over 30 °C. That theoretically means that while it's in the truck being transported through a Swedish winter or an Egyptian summer the drug is going to lose efficacy. The same if you leave it in your car to go shopping on the way back from the pharmacy. This is a truly worrying problem as I've been in Maracaibo, Venezuela for periods when the temperature never dropped below 30 °C even at night and most people can't afford air conditioning. A drug that is so fragile that it requires constant air conditioning and/or heating is massively unsuited for Third World use.

A little bit of good news has come out of the westward migration of infected wild birds from Western China that have since arrived in Europe. The type of H5N1 they carry has not been affected by China's overprescription of the human pharmaceuticals Symmetrel (*amantadine hydrochloride*) and Flumadine (*rimantadine hydrochloride*) on millions of poultry, which has caused some forms of the virus to develop a resistance. Symmetrel and Flumadine are considerably less expensive than Tamiflu or Relenza and far more readily available. Should the pandemic issue from these Symmetrel/Flumadine-sensitive strains, then these would become the drugs of choice. However, they are far from perfect either.

Symmetrel's usual adult dosage is 200 milligrams per day. Yet, deaths have been recorded at overdoses of just five times this amount. Also, this drug has been linked to suicide attempts (and successes) among people who both did and did not previously have any history of mental illness – and nobody seems to know why. There are also reports of a whole plethora of unsavoury side effects, such as disorientation, confusion, depression, personality changes, agitation, aggressive behaviour, hallucinations, paranoia, other psychotic reactions, somnolence, insomnia and increased epileptic seizures.

Its cousin Flumadine has not been linked to suicides at this time, but it presents a whole cornucopia of side effects, such as increased epileptic seizures, impaired concentration, insomnia, dizziness, headache, fatigue, nervousness, nausea, vomiting, anorexia, dry mouth, abdominal pain and general body aches.

Another problem with both of these drugs is that when you take them, between 10 per cent and 30 per cent of the virus you shed to the outside world is resistant to them. That's what happened in the Chinese instance when they medicated their poultry with these. They did it so much and for so long that all the virus in that area became resistant. In a human pandemic situation, it is expected that if these drugs were used at the beginning of the pandemic, the majority of the virus circulating just weeks later would be resistant. So these drugs may be just a short term, early pandemic stopgap in the best case.

*

Some late-breaking reports indicate that a 'cocktail' of Tamiflu used in connection with Symmetrel may act more effectively than either drug alone. While Tamiflu targets the N mushrooms, Symmetrel is effective against a different part of the (Symmetrel-sensitive forms of) H5N1 virus called M2. As mentioned above, at the time of writing most forms of H5N1 winging their way towards Europe and North America in wild birds were still Symmetrel-susceptible, so if that forms the basis for the pandemic, the Tamiflu–Symmetrel cocktail could be a useful pharmaceutical weapon. However, there are still many forms of H5N1 that are fully resistant to Symmetrel and these forms could find their way around the world on much faster wings – those of jet-liners.

The National Institute for Clinical Excellence (NICE) in the UK issues guidelines for the use of pharmaceuticals and medical procedures. Here is what they have to say about the H5N1 antivirals:

> Symmetrel is not recommended for post-exposure prophylaxis, seasonal prophylaxis or treatment of influenza.
> Tamiflu and Relenza are not recommended for seasonal prophylaxis against influenza.
>
> Tamiflu and Relenza are not recommended for post-exposure prophylaxis or treatment of otherwise healthy individuals with influenza.
>
> Tamiflu is recommended for post-exposure prophylaxis in at-risk adults and adolescents over 13 years who are not effectively protected by the influenza vaccine and who can start treatment within 48 hours of close contact with someone suffering from influenza-like illness. Prophylaxis is also recommended for residents in care establishments

who can start treatment within 48 hours if the illness is present in the establishment.

Tamiflu and Relenza are recommended to treat at-risk adults who can start treatment within 48 hours of the onset of symptoms. Relenza is recommended for at-risk children who can start treatment within the same period.

These guidelines basically obviate and, to some extent, contradict the common practice and established clinical use of these drugs. Tamiflu and Relenza's strongest point may be in the very use of 'seasonal prophylaxis', or taking the drug daily when the pandemic hits your geographical area. By waiting for a day or two after there has been confirmed contact with H5N1, especially given the fact that people in the early stages of H5N1 infection don't even know themselves that they are contagious is ridiculously late.

It may or may not be fortunate that very few physicians pay any attention. Dr Michael Dixon, chairman of the NHS Alliance, states: 'The fact that some NICE guidelines are ignored is not necessarily a bad thing. NICE sends out a set of guidelines every other week. It comes in the form of a thick booklet. I have enough of these booklets to wallpaper my entire surgery. I and many other doctors simply don't have the time to read it.'

Now that we have an overview of the antiviral drugs that are available and their effectiveness or lack thereof, the decision you have to make is whether you want to build up your own personal stockpile. Tamiflu, Relenza, Symmetrel and Flumadine are generally available by prescription only. I strongly doubt that your local doctor is going to be willing to write scripts for several hundred pills for each member of your family as most doctors will only prescribe ten Tamiflus at a time and usually restrict their use for when flu symptoms are present. Doctors do not generally prescribe for prophylaxis use and you will probably find it quite difficult to convince your doctor to do so.

If you have decided that stockpiling is the way to go, then you may have no choice but to turn to online pharmacies. The online pharmacy industry has received a generally bad rap in the press, and much of it is well deserved. There were many fly-by-night operators that set up shop in the early days of the industry and sold stale-dated, improper or even outright-counterfeit medications. Some of these sharks are still out there, but there has been a movement in the last couple of years towards industry self-regulation and at least three international online pharmacy accreditation and standards-enforcement organisations have been established. I strongly advise that if you choose to purchase pharmaceuticals from online pharmacies you check with one of these standards organisations first and order only from their member pharmacies in good standing. The Resources section at the end of this book has extensive contact information for the three standards organisations and many of the top online pharmacies.

You will find that most of the larger online pharmacies are located in Canada and in the province of Manitoba specifically. The industry seemed to find its original base there due to various legislative loopholes in the provincial laws and today it still mostly resides there and in the province of Alberta. There are many other online pharmacies around the world. It is hard to think of any major nation that doesn't have at least a couple. You may find that ordering from your own nation's online pharmacies may avoid some costly shipping charges and customs hassles. However, different countries have different regulations regarding dispensing pharmaceuticals and ordering locally can sometimes be more trouble than it saves. I have only ever placed orders with Canadian online pharmacies and have yet to experience any problems whatsoever. The Canadians seem to be the world standard at this time, but this may change in the future. You may want to note that receiving prescription pharmaceuticals across international borders may present various legal problems depending on what jurisdiction you live in, so you may be well advised to check with your local pharmaceutical board or customs office as to the regulations that apply in your country.

The question that has bedevilled the online pharmacy industry from day one has been the problem with prescriptions. There are some fully reputable online pharmacies that will sell you absolutely anything in any quantity you want, simply on your self-declaration that you need the drug. There are others that have varying levels of confirmation before they fill the prescription and may ask you to fax them a copy of the prescription or in other ways be in contact with your doctor. Some even ask you to fill out an online questionnaire and will only prescribe what their pharmacist deems reasonable given your answers.

Again, the choice is yours. You can easily find a reputable online pharmacy to fill your order with no questions asked except your credit card number and shipping address. If you feel that this is the best option, then you should use your best judgement. Some people will only want to fill a prescription online that was given to them by their doctor, which then begs the question of why go through the online international shipping process at all. You may find that, in many cases, the savings on the retail price of the drug get eaten up by shipping and other charges anyway. Given the fact that Tamiflu may be in fearfully short supply for years, you may find that the online pharmacies are the only ones that have stocks of the Roche drug. Note that inventory levels fluctuate daily and, at the time of writing, Tamiflu is becoming painfully scarce and the prices are spiking upwards. The effect of Roche's temporary embargo on selling to various distributors will be that these pharmacies will have to source their Tamiflu farther afield which raises their costs. Be warned that you may have to do a lot of emailing before you find an online pharmacy that has Tamiflu in stock and is willing to sell it to you at a non-extortionate price.

Here comes the warning label: Tamiflu, Relenza, Symmetrel and Flumadine all have serious side effects and can be extremely dangerous if not taken under the advice and supervision of a physician. Your own personal stockpile could turn out to cause you more physical problems than it could cure. I do not advise purchasing prescription drugs without a prescription.

Having said that, I don't practise what I preach and I have a significant stockpile of fresh Tamiflu in my home. Draw whatever conclusions you like.

Listings on where to obtain the products discussed in this section can be found in the Resources.

CHAPTER 10

The Race to Make Not Enough of the Wrong Vaccine

If there s a vaccine in time that actually works, get it!

A vaccine is a formulation that is injected into healthy people in the expectation that they will develop immunity towards a specific disease. Flu vaccines are made from the virus that causes that particular disease. Unlike homeopathy, which uses the cause of a particular disease in virtually infinite dilution in the hope of curing it, the viruses used in flu vaccine are inactivated or segmented so that they cannot make you ill, but instead your body will develop an immunity by its antibodies against it for when the real thing comes along. Once the vaccine triggers the formation of antibodies that will stop the virus, and your body is able to maintain that at a high-enough level, you can be infected with that virus but it won't make you ill.

In most cases, the vaccine works as designed and keeps you from getting the disease caused by the virus. In a few cases, some viruses manage to outsmart the antibodies, or the inactivated virus in the vaccine itself is not quite inactivated enough and gives you the disease that it was supposed to give you immunity from.

The Race to Make Not Enough

The recent history of flu vaccines has been anything but stellar. In 2003–2004 there was an increased demand for vaccine as the flu season came early and hit hard. The demand could not be met and severe shortages developed. The flu season of 2004–2005 saw a contamination of the vaccine produced by Chiron wipe out half the existing stocks.

Note that these problems were during more or less 'normal flu seasons', which are to a pandemic what a roller skate is to Michael Schumacher's Ferrari. It is quite obvious to all the experts that the demand of any vaccine will far outstrip supply during a pandemic, perhaps by as much as 500 to 1.

That allows for the expectation that there will actually be a vaccine that works against H5N1, which is proving to be a difficult target to hit. The reasons for this are many and varied. Vaccine production is a complex subject and far outside the scope of this book, but let's suffice it to say that, at the time of writing, the specific characteristics of the virus found in wild birds migrating from the Qinghai region of western China are significantly different from the virus that is being used to develop the pandemic vaccine. The prototype for the vaccine is based on a strain of H5N1 that has been 'reverse-genetically engineered'. At this point no one knows if this vaccine will be effective at all against whatever strain finally triggers the pandemic. Unfortunately it is that very different form of the virus which is being carried from China through Russia and, as I write this, into Europe by these migrating birds.

The vaccine that is being developed and hailed as the saviour against H5N1 requires at least 180 micrograms of virus (or maybe more) to get even a mild response from the human antibodies. This may seem like an infinitesimal amount, but when you consider that some existing vaccines such as the trivalent only use 15 micrograms, 12 times as much 'raw' virus is an immense amount to produce for the vaccine.

It's still not quite that easy to produce the vaccine against H5N1, even if we can cope with the large amounts required and shift to the current strain invading Europe through the wild bird migrations. Setting up production on such a global scale may take years. Although some newer technologies are in the works, most vaccine development is still performed in fertile chicken eggs, exactly like a century ago. H5N1 has shown a remarkable ability to mutate very quickly. It keeps changing its characteristics through its antigenic shifts, evolving from one form to another. Even if we were successful in isolating this particular form of the virus that exists in these late summer 2005 wild birds, it might take up to eight months to have sufficient, tested vaccine stocks to start immunising people. And by then, the H5N1 virus may very well have mutated into another form that is much more dangerous to humans and much more resistant to the antibodies stimulated by the vaccine.

In clay pigeon shooting it is good practice to lead ahead of the flying clay disc with your rifle's sight so that the bullet reaches where the clay will be at the moment of impact, not where it is when the bullet is actually fired. Imagine if you were shooting clay pigeons that could change direction randomly and much faster than the bullet could reach them. You could shoot pretty well wherever you wanted in the sky and you would have the same, very slight, random chance of hitting any of them.

The Race to Make Not Enough

That is not unlike what it is like to create a vaccine for H5N1. You have to hope that the clay pigeon will keep flying in a straight line, since you cannot possibly create a vaccine that forecasts where the clay will be by the time the bullet hits it, which in the case of vaccine can be just short of a year.

The biggest problem is that once H5N1 becomes a fully human-to-human transmissible disease, it will start spreading through the population like wildfire. It could be the current Qinghai-originating strain, or it could be the one that the vaccines have been patterned upon, or it could be something very different. Nobody can know in advance. We will have to wait until it happens. Unfortunately, once it's happened, the pandemic will spread much faster than the vaccine can be created, tested and distributed. The first wave of the pandemic could be through in two or three months. Conventional vaccines can take three or four times this long to become available.

Once they become available, if they are actually in time to help stem the pandemic, the problem becomes how to produce enough of it; 180 micrograms or more of virus vaccine presents enormous problems in production. The best estimate right now is for 75 million doses of vaccine as a legitimate maximum target. We have over 6.5 billion people on this planet right now. At best the vaccine will only be available for 1 out of every 86 of us. And it could quite believably be far less.

Governments all over the world have ordered H5N1 vaccine. Well, at least they've tendered for it. They can't really order what doesn't yet exist. But no matter how much they order or even end up getting, they will only be able to vaccinate a tiny percentage of their population. US President Bush's November 2005 'Super-Flu Policy' calls for $1.2 billion to purchase enough doses of any eventual H5N1 vaccine to protect 20 million Americans, or 7 per cent of the US population, and $2.8 billion to speed the development of vaccines as new strains emerge. The UK government has ordered 2 million doses of the vaccine. Furthermore the experimental vaccine trial was based on administering two doses plus a booster shot. Therefore, the 2 million doses may end up vaccinating only 650,000 people. Similar situations exist in all the other countries that have ordered vaccine. Germany will be able to vaccinate less than a million of its citizens, and Spain less than half a million. Presented with the problem that most people will not be able to get that vaccine, governments will have to decide which people will receive it. In almost every country those that will be allocated the vaccine are strictly medical and governmental personnel, and if there is any left (and there won't be), then it will be for the highest risk demographic group.

We all have the stereotype in mind of the perfect citizen: altruistic, community-minded and self-sacrificing for the common good. Unfortunately, I'm seeing fewer and fewer of these people around. Wherever I look, I'm seeing a shadow of opportunism, egotism and disregard for society surfacing all around me. There are many people I know personally who faced with a situation such as this would simply march down to the local surgery or pharmacy with a crowbar and do whatever is necessary to get the vaccine for themselves and their family. I don't know if I would go quite that far, but the prospect of being given an opportunity to live strictly based on whether or not you get a government pay cheque is not one that I care to face. I don't know if I could idly stand by as the pandemic was ravaging the country knowing that the orderly at the hospital has the vaccine but I don't. And I don't know how many others would have that wherewithal either.

As much as I respect the medical personnel, I truly wonder whether the doctor or nurse that receives the vaccine is not going to sneak a dose out under their jacket to their child at home. Could you possibly blame them for attempting that? Under the same circumstances, many of us would do the same.

This is one of those rare cases where medical policy crosses over into social policy. I cannot imagine how anyone can justify administering a potentially life-saving vaccine to one and a half per cent of its population, leaving the rest to fend for themselves. I'm well aware that the expectation of the 2 million vaccines is all that can be hoped for, and that it would be a truly best case scenario if we were actually to get that many doses that were effective. Regardless, it is triggers like these that start the avalanche of massive social unrest and civil disobedience with results that are impossible to predict.

The vaccine prospect is a damned-if-you-do-and-damned-if-you-don't scenario. There is no way you can win. If the vaccine works, then you probably won't get it. If the vaccine doesn't work, then nobody gets it anyway. From an overall social standpoint it might be better if there is no vaccine, then we all get to suffer in equality. The prospect of a 2-million strong New Mandarin class being given the gift of life to the exclusion of everyone else presents prospects for social upheaval that are too grim to contemplate.

Since the modern world is the interconnected labyrinth that it is today, you can rest assured that there will be a thriving online and black-market commerce in the vaccine.

Some will be fresh and effective, some will be outdated and weak, and some will be sugar water. Regardless, there will be people paying hundreds or thousands of pounds or much much more to get their hands on the real thing. To a man living in a grand manor house with two new Mercedes in the garage and a healthy stock portfolio, what is £50,000/$90,000 to ensure the health and safety of his family? A minor blip on his financial radar. He probably lost that much on Marconi, Nortel or Enron stock. To the rest of us it's an impossible price to pay. To a Third World worker it could be more than the yearly income of his entire village.

Faced with financial incentives of this magnitude, who can say that the vaccine manufacturers can ensure that all of the vaccine will find its way into the 'proper' channels? When the lab worker who earns less than £10/$18 per hour faces the prospect of sneaking a vial or two in his pocket (or worse anatomical place) and netting a few tens of thousands of pounds, do you really think they're going to leave the vial in the factory? Or do you think that the security guard who earns £8/$14.40 per hour is going to stop them? Quite unlikely. Most likely they'll split the vaccine and sneak it all out. Those people are going to take that vaccine, administer it to their spouses and kids, and then sell off the rest for a substantial amount of money. It's going to happen. And it's going to happen over and over again. It's human nature.

Let's not even mention what will happen when gangsters get wind of the fact that a couple of little bottles of liquid can be sold for tens of thousands of pounds, at a profit margin much higher than any narcotic currently on the street. With their pre-existing underground international distribution networks, the switch from coke to vaccine will be virtually instantaneous, giving rise to the capitalistic paradigm of the 21st century: 'You wanna live? How much money you got?'

There have been some glimmers of hope to break this uninterrupted curtain of gloom, in that at the end of the summer of 2005 there were some reports of a possible vaccine that targets a different part of the H5N1 virus, one that does not mutate from form to form. That would be extremely welcome news; it would provide, instead of a single bullet, a whole shotgun full of pellets that would spray the entire sky to hit the clay (viral) target. However, even if such a vaccine can be produced, there are still the same limitations as with all the other types. The dream of producing enough vaccine to keep over 6.5 billion people completely safe from H5N1 will remain a dream for some time. Again, no one can know the future and there may be some tremendous Nobel-Prize-winning breakthrough in some lab somewhere in the world right now that will allow for vaccine manufacture and distribution in a completely new fashion. We may be able to swiftly and fully vaccinate every man, woman and child in the world with a supremely effective H5N1 vaccine, relegating this dark killer to the scrap heap of medical history along with smallpox and polio. A development of this scale would most certainly be a cause for great rejoicing. We can only hope that the nightmare of the pandemic doesn't reach us until the dream does.

CHAPTER 11

What Governments Can Do Today

How the pandemic could rip the world apart

The riots began in Rome at the height of the flu pandemic, when a march along Viale Regina Elena by the trade unions CGIL, CISL and UIL to protest corruption in the distribution of Bird Flu vaccine by the Italian Government turned ugly. The demonstrators were confronted by over 10,000 medical personnel demanding that they have first rights to the limited vaccine stocks. In the resultant melee, over 1,000 demonstrators and bystanders were injured and more than 100 were killed. This was only the beginning of the casualties as several hundred more deaths and thousands of injuries were caused when the trade unionists turned to Viale del Policlinico and burned Rome's largest hospital, the Umberto I Polyclinic, in an attempt to loot the vaccine within. The Italian Armed Forces working with the Carabinieri managed to arrest several thousand demonstrators and the Italian Prime Minister declared the Capital under martial law.

Within a week other major European cities including Lyon, Barcelona, Lisbon and Zagreb had all witnessed similar events. The worst rioting was in Athens where angry mobs looted hospitals and pharmacies throughout the city. The accompanying runaway arson blazes, fuelled by a strong northerly meltemi wind, destroyed several hundred city blocks stretching from the Attiko Alsos all the way to the Parliament and Panathenian Stadium. The Parthenon, Agora, Herodeion and many other world heritage temples were destroyed or irreparably damaged.

These incidents turned to a continent-wide crisis when the summit of EU leaders in Brussels called to discuss the international riots was firebombed by crowds demanding vaccine. Most European heads of state, foreign secretaries and chief medical officers were killed or severely injured. This simultaneous decapitation of most of the EU leadership was swiftly followed by runaway rioting and looting that left large portions of Manchester, Naples, Munich, Copenhagen, Prague and Cork in ruins.

Demonstrations spread across the United States as well, with major riots and looting in Miami, Cleveland, Philadelphia and Los Angeles. Several major hospitals and health facilities in Houston were raided, with local law enforcement officials blaming it on the 'criminal refugees from the New Orleans floods'.

The provisional European Union President announced from the intensive care ward of the Belgian University Hospital that the EU had formally called upon NATO troops to enforce an international curfew on all member states and to restore calm across a burning continent. Even the resolve of this massive military force was attenuated by the incapacitation of over 40 per cent of its officers and soldiers to the rampaging pandemic, as the strife and the flu spread to every major city in Europe. With Western governments unable to bolster their traditional allies, much of Israel was overrun by Palestinian and Jordanian troops.

Beat the Flu

The Israeli Prime Minister gave the invaders 24 hours to leave or threatened to restore Israel's borders by 'the nuclear option'.

This is definitely a worst-case scenario. It is not very likely that the hundreds of millions of otherwise rational and sane citizens of the European Union would turn into rampaging raiders stopping at nothing, including looting and burning their own communities, just to get their hands on a vial of vaccine or a dose of antiviral and that it would lead to nuclear strikes. However, the bottom line is that it does not take an overwhelming event to spark violent madness in a mob. It can happen anywhere and at any time. There is virtually no one alive today who lived through the 1918 pandemic, so we cannot estimate how people today will react to such a pervasive threat to public health and how they will judge the reaction of their governments and health authorities. When your family and friends are dying all around you, it takes great self-control not to strike back at a government and a society that can be seen as having failed to take decisive steps to prevent this tragedy.

In September of 1918, the US War Department found its troops so debilitated by the Spanish Flu that they could not put down the riots that were flaring up around the country due to the public hysteria caused by the pandemic. These riots were not so much against the governmental health services' reaction or lack thereof, but just born and fuelled by the hysteria caused by people watching their communities die around them. In 1918 most people understood that medical science had not developed to a point where government action could have stopped the pandemic in its tracks. In the generations since, that perception has changed. We have become accustomed to medical miracles.

Most citizens of developed nations have a righteous expectation that in return for their taxes their government will protect them against massive threats to the public health.

The tragic September 11 attacks on the US claimed less than 3,000 lives and sparked an expenditure of several hundreds of billions of dollars through military action in Afghanistan and Iraq as well as expensive international security measures. Yet now we are facing the prospect of losing more than 100,000 times this many people. The unfortunate truth is that world governments are stumbling around in the myopic process of ordering antivirals that will be backordered for years and vaccines that may not arrive until well after the pandemic has struck and be ineffective when they finally are ready.

The plan for immediate action rather than waiting in vain for a miracle cure

What is done is done, and governments all over the world are slowly waking up to the reality that the storm is at the door and they are woefully unprepared. What can the governments of the world do today that will have an effect upon this modern plague?

Here is a list of things that can be done by the governments, and some of them might surprise you.

1) Engage in a serious and immediate educational media blitz. Shatter the preconception of the public that this is just another bunch of doomsayer crackpot scientists trying to secure bigger research grants. Bring the issue to the forefront through every means of communication available, even if hours a day of broadcast time has to be appropriated and redirected from tepid escapism to this critical issue. Run

continuous programming demonstrating proper hygiene and infection-prevention techniques.

2) Set up a domestic version of the US Peace Corps, where thousands of people are sent out throughout the nation to train communities on how to keep themselves safe through common-sense techniques, such as those illustrated in this book.

3) Issue N-95 respirators, ample supplies of alcohol hand sanitisers and infection control instructions to every household in the country at no charge.

4) Prepare the economy for a prolonged shutdown. Introduce a 50 per cent subsidy to the retail cost of selected canned, preserved and dried foods and plain bottled water. Remove all duties, excise and sales taxes on a list of essential products from electrical generators to wind-up radios. Apply 25 per cent of all personal income and corporate taxes to a fund to help families and businesses rebuild after the pandemic.

5) Make up the cost to the national budget of the above plans by slashing the defence budget and repatriating troops serving in foreign countries. Issue each officer and soldier a Level-A bio-protective suit and retrain them to administer pandemic education and emergency services.

6) Establish an Idea Grant Programme where any citizen can suggest some way to increase flu safety and receive a substantial grant to research and implement it at the community level.

7) Restrict entrance to the country only to returning citizens for the duration. Test them all for H5N1 at the entry port. Quarantine and treat any testing positive.

*

Interestingly, none of these suggestions involve buying drugs, vaccines or even investing in medical research projects. Limited advances can be derived from government involvement in science in such a short timeframe. If researchers do create a truly effective drug that can be administered in time to the entire population, by all means the government should purchase it at going market rate. Otherwise, we should concentrate on the social aspects of the pandemic rather than the medical if there is no way to stimulate a breakthrough for the treatment of the entire population.

This is an immensely controversial plan that flies in the face of the conventional wisdom that calls for medical science to pull magical bunnies out of a hat and save the world on an ongoing basis. I believe that it is time that governments realise that, just like HIV/AIDS, H5N1 is a human crisis even more than a medical one. The damage to the social fabric of a nation that can be caused by a ravaging pandemic is immense, especially when there is no hope of treating more than an infinitesimal percentage of the population. The onus must shift to preparation and survivability.

Governments can certainly commandeer significant resources when it is so required. In late September 2005, facing a then-small outbreak of H5N1, the Indonesian government announced that they would use force to take people suspected of being infected with the virus into hospital. It seems that long-cherished civil rights are summarily dispensed with when faced with potential pandemics. And that is not altogether wrong. H5N1 represents a tremendous challenge to public health.

When I wrote an early draft of this book, several of the first readers chided me for my bombastic and unlikely conclusions. Entire countries couldn't simply close their borders, they remarked. It was next to impossible. Yet, reality has a way of becoming more unlikely than fiction and Australia recently announced that in the case of a pandemic they would seal off the entire border of the island continent for the duration: nobody enters until the pandemic wave has passed. Australia's geographical isolation makes such a policy feasible, but this is not a practical option for most countries. It could easily be implemented by Japan, the UK and Ireland, Iceland, Malta, Cyprus, Madagascar, Sri Lanka, the Philippines, New Zealand, much of Indonesia and many Caribbean and South Pacific islands, but most countries share porous land borders with their neighbours. Some parts of the Canadian/US Border have only one enforcement agent per 50 kilometres.

Many of the world's countries have been preparing contingency plans for the pandemic. Most of these are rather similar and focus on accelerating availability and distribution of antiviral drugs and vaccines; health screening, including at entry ports; quarantines; and restrictions on travel and public events. Some countries such as the UK have coherent policy programmes in place that are implementable at short notice.

Michael Osterholm of the University of Minnesota, in advising the Bush administration for what has been called 'the super-plan against the super-flu', has stated:

> Understand that a lot of the things we need to do to prepare are not related to magic bullets. How to provide food supplies, everyday medical care for people who don't have the super-flu, basic utilities and even security must be part of the plan. In this day and age of a global economy, with just-in-time delivery, no surge capacity and international

supply chains – those things are very difficult to do for a week, let alone for 12 to 18 months of what will be a very tough time.

The United States has already announced that they would call in the military to enforce a form of germ martial law, empowering them to forcefully quarantine entire communities or even states. Although the militaristic element was found by some observers in other countries to be overkill, I have to admit that it may well come to the stage where this type of national response may be required.

CHAPTER 12

Surviving the Pandemic Financially

How to secure your investments through a pandemic

We live in a money-driven society, thus the survival of thousands is equated in some circles with the impact on the Profits and Losses sheet. It is inevitable that there will be many people who regard this upcoming pandemic as a threat to their bottom line more than to their health.

There are various levels of personal and business investment and, although it is well-nigh impossible to accurately gauge the effect of a pandemic that no one knows when will hit or how hard, there are some guidelines to determine how some of these investments are likely to fare.

In light of statements by health-care officials that the pandemic could have the hardest impact on people between 20 and 40 (as in 1918), the most economically productive age group, many financial experts lined up their estimates of what impact the pandemic could have on business. Leading business analyst firm Standard & Poor had these forecasts:

It could mean a substantial reduction of global trade. That could lead to new energy shortages and affect a wide variety of imports and exports, particularly manufactured goods from the Pacific Basin.

David Braverman, Vice President, portfolio services group

Casinos and hotels would likely experience lower demand depending on their location. Cruise-ship operators and sporting events would lose business if people avoided enclosed places where large groups of people are typically in close proximity.

Tom Graves, Analyst, equity analysis group

Increased telecommuting would benefit IP service providers based in Asia, and traditional wireline and wireless carriers.

Ken Leon, Analyst, telecom analysis group

The Netherlands-based international ING bank warned:

large swathes of economic activity could simply cease. A realistic scenario might involve GDP declines of tens of percent. We believe that fear of infection leading to drastically altered behaviour would result in the greatest economic damage. Investors would likely shun equities and corporate bonds. Although economic activity would slump, inflation might well soar due to the interruption of supplies and loss of production.

Michael Lewis, head of commodities research at Deutsche Bank, said:

This would be an extreme negative shock to the world economy. You'd see equity markets unravelling everywhere as people began to think through the implications.

Olusoji Adeyi, public health co-ordinator at the World Bank, said:

> Health care workers might be dying in large numbers, therefore the health services as we know them might cease to function. Supply and distribution chains might break down. Even if one country were able to hunker down and immunise all its residents effectively, what about the knock-on effect of the potential global economic meltdown?

The USA's Pandemic Influenza Strategic Plan stated the virus could lead to food and fuel shortages and power blackouts. Schools would be shut, a quarter of the work-force would refuse to go to work, and there might be riots at vaccination centres.

Canada's Conference Board stated in an October 2005 report that a major pandemic would 'throw the world into a sudden and possibly dramatic global recession.'

The Canadian investment house BMO Nesbitt Burns, part of the international Bank of Montreal group, issued a prophetic pandemic report in August 2005. This report was stark in its appraisal of the overwhelming global economic impact of a pandemic, and much of the information and projections contained in this chapter are extrapolations from this report and the albeit 'educated guesses' or musings from other financial experts.

The true 'bottom line' is that the world's economy has developed significantly from the last major flu pandemic almost a century ago, thus very little guidance can be derived from history. No one can truly comprehend how an interconnected speed-of-light global economy will fare under worldwide pandemic conditions. In such an unprecedented global catastrophe, the best computer models are inadequate and the most insightful Wall Street guru's opinion is worth barely more than the man on the street so these recommendations are best taken with a grain of salt.

A Chinese curse says 'may you live in interesting times' and the times ahead could definitely be interesting. However, no one knows exactly how interesting. It is impossible to gauge today how hard the pandemic is going to hit. It may be widespread but very mild, or it may be localised to a particular geographical area. In the other extreme it could ravage every country in the world killing hundreds of millions of people. For the purposes of this analysis, I've broken down these possibilities to three levels of potential pandemic:

Low: This model is based upon forecasts of 250 million infected and 25 million dead worldwide in a single, three-month flu season.

Medium: This model is based upon forecasts of one billion infected and 100 million dead worldwide in a single, six-month flu season.

High: This is the apocalyptic model. It forecasts over five billion infected and deaths upwards of half a billion people in multiple waves stretching over a year.

Investments, Savings and Pensions

Stock and bond prices go up and down every minute of every day to reflect the perception of how well a company is doing. In actual fact, there seems to be no precise correlations between real tangible asset values and valuations based on market sentiment. That's why a company like General Motors or Ford that owns dozens of multi-billion-dollar plants all over the world, has hundreds of thousands of employees, and has indisputable tangible worth, has a lower overall value on the stock market than a company like Google that effectively is nothing more than an ethereal website that does little more than just point to other websites. So irrational is this system, that the current market value of Google is more than three times General Motors and Ford combined.

We all remember the various booms such as the 'dot com' bubble where millionaires were being made overnight. The Dow Jones Industrial Average, the world's leading index, was rising like a helium balloon. Some financial soothsayers were predicting 20,000, 30,000 or even six-figure levels in the near future. Then a couple of planes flew into buildings and the Dow Jones flatlined at around 10,000 and hasn't budged significantly since.

How would the Dow, FTSE, All Ordinaries and other indexes react to a true worldwide catastrophe? No one has a crystal ball in cases like this, therefore it is quite impossible to predict accurately. Most analysts look back to 1929 to determine the structure of a market crash, but so much has changed since that time that it is an unreliable model. There is no hard and fast forecast for what could happen during a global flu pandemic.

Keep in mind that in a typical influenza season with 300,000 people out of over 300 million in the US falling seriously ill, the total cost to the economy is $14.58 billion, which is like taking out the entire Gross Domestic Product (GDP) of Panama. A 10 per cent infection rate in the population during a pandemic could cost the UK the GDP of South Africa, cost Germany the GDP of Poland and the US the entire GDP of the 1.3 billion people in China.

Stock markets

Now, let's look at how the stock markets would react to the Low and Medium scenarios (the High scenario is too devastating to consider) to show how various equities would perform in these situations. These again, are just guesses, as the greatest Wall Street gurus don't really know any more than anyone else:

Low: Service and retail companies would be most severely affected as people would tend to stay indoors and avoid unnecessary shopping trips. These companies could see an overall 20 per cent drop in share price, with many marginal companies folding altogether. The industrial sector would be hit by low employee turnout, resulting in curtailed productivity of approximately 10 per cent, which could result in a share price drop of about 15 per cent. These drops would have a knock-on effect through the economy and most leading indicators could fall by approximately 25 per cent. A Dow Jones in the 7,000s is likely (it has been between 10,000 and 10,500 since 9/11). The worst performing companies would be in non-essential products and services such as high-priced clothing, cosmetics, jewellery, sports cars, Rolexes, high-end electronics, etc. Potential winners would be food, energy and utility companies, as prices are certain to rise in these segments and would represent the wisest share investment. The overall market would not be expected to fully recover to pre-pandemic balance for at least 18 to 24 months.

Medium: This much higher level of absenteeism and loss of consumer confidence caused by legitimate global safety fears would have a notably stronger effect on the worldwide economy. Service, retail and manufacturing would be a washout, with share prices falling 70 per cent or more. The Dow could drop below 3,000 unless it was drastically restructured to jettison the many failing blue-chip companies. Many global brands could not survive this shakeout and would disappear or be bought out at bargain basement prices by raiders. Internet stocks could skyrocket as much of the world's population that can afford it would turn to electronic communication and commerce as it shuns face-to-face activities for fear of contagion. The new successes could be companies that deliver irradiated or otherwise sterilised food and supplies to the upper echelon of householders. Transportation would be severely hit as people avoid travel of any kind. Airlines would be hardest hit, many fatally. Energy prices would skew significantly as the demand for motor fuels diminishes but electricity demands rise. The overall market would not be expected to fully recover to pre-pandemic balance for at least four to six years.

Individual savings

Individual savings could be hit hard as well. The rock-hard solidity of the banking system could crumble under the impact of a global pandemic:

Low: The effect of a Dow in the 7,000s will hit the banks hardest as residential and commercial estate values deflate and commercial loans go sour by the millions. Even though the banks are covered by various Federal Deposit Insurances, these funds don't have the reserve capacity to bail out a number of large bank failures all at once. These fears may lead to a run on the banks that will help to push some of the weaker ones over the brink surprisingly quickly.

Medium: The banks are clearly the most vulnerable sector (next to discretionary products and services) and savings will suffer in the inevitable runs. The exposure of the banks to a collapse is in the trillions of pounds or dollars.

Pensions

Many people depend on their pensions to carry them through old age. Yet pensions are very susceptible to a pandemic's economic impact as well:

Low: A pension is only worth what you can get back from it in 'real terms' and that is where the problem lies when a pandemic's economic effects are factored in. To simply believe the pension fund managers when they state that their investments are indexed to inflation does not absolve you of responsibility to determine just how safe that fund is when subjected to global crises. It is highly recommended that you sit down with your pension fund representative before the pandemic hits, and determine what your pension prospects are, should there be significant economic disruptions ahead. You may be shocked at the lack of preparation your fund manager has taken to safeguard your pension.

Medium: Pensions would have little or no value at this point. Many pensions invest heavily into the stock markets and the Dow plummeting into the 3,000s and the FTSE in triple digits would see the collapse of almost every single pension fund in the world. The best possible pension investment in this scenario is investing in family. That may sound ridiculous, but when you consider it for a moment, it's not as silly as it may seem. If the monetary assurances of sufficient funding during your twilight years were to evaporate, then you would have nothing to fall back on to take care of your needs. Except family! An extended family on good terms with each other will assure that the elderly members are taken care of, sheltered, fed and made as comfortable as possible. The younger members will work to earn a living and they will share their income to sustain the elders. That is the way that families have worked for thousands of years, and it is only a recent phenomenon to leave the elderly to fend for themselves alone. By revitalising this traditional family structure, you may find that there is a much greater benefit than just making sure that food is on the table and wood in the hearth. You may find that it is an alternative to an independent, albeit lonely old age, surrounded by the warmth and security of family. So now may be the time to build bridges with your family wherever they may be. They may turn out to be your saving grace.

The value of varied investments in a pandemic era

There are countless other investments available, but none of them offer any specific security in a pandemic era. Investment-grade art will be worthless as it offers no tangible benefit and is primarily of interest to the rarefied connoisseur, who will likely be caught up in other, more immediate interests. The same applies to collectibles, toys, antiques and other overvalued items. They are only worth what the aficionado is willing to pay. Wine is an interesting investment since, unlike art and other collectibles, you can actually drink it. However, at the prices that some vintages are fetching, you could buy the entire stock of the local corner shop.

Again, we are looking into these investments as potential insurance policies for the inevitable economic paroxysms that will accompany a pandemic. If the pandemic is Low, then things will get shaken up a bit and then settle back down soon enough. But if it goes to Medium Severity and upwards, the effects will be so far-reaching and pervasive that it will mark a turning point in human history.

Classic cars as an investment are also not recommended in a pandemic era. Although there have been times in the recent past where classic car prices have shot through the roof, with people paying millions for classics in concours condition, there is no indication that those valuations will survive a pandemic, especially a Medium range or stronger one. Transportation bottlenecks will accelerate the death of the internal combustion engine as fuels simply cease to be available. We have to consider that even in the Medium scenario, we have one billion people infected, of which 10 per cent will die. Those rates of infection are so massive that the vast majority of people on Earth will take every possible opportunity to not venture outside their homes for fear of contagion. When people are living in a fearful environment like that, the idea of blasting down country lanes in a convertible Jaguar somehow loses its sheen.

There seems to be one investment that has integral and virtually eternal lustre. From the times of the earliest civilisations, people all over the world have been transfixed by the apparently magical properties of gold. Egyptian pharaohs were buried in heavily gilded tombs. In later times, much of the exploration of the New World was driven by the desire to find El Dorado, the mythical city built of solid gold.

Investment opportunities for gold include buying equities in gold mining companies, or mutual funds that invest across a spectrum of gold stocks. However, many people prefer to have, touch, feel and hold their gold, therefore gold bullion or coins are very popular.

These days, gold seems to retain its value, regardless of political or economic uncertainty, and in some cases outperforms any other investment. Gold's value tends to rise whenever confidence in the economy is shaken and a pandemic will likely trigger a rise in gold at first. Indeed, if the pandemic remains in the Low scenario range, then gold may be an excellent investment. It is not outlandish to expect that by the end of a Low pandemic season, gold would have retested its all-time highs of just under £500/$900 per ounce. The problem with gold is that it is intrinsically an abstract value. Nothing much of indispensable value can be done with gold. It is primarily an adornment and indicator of value rather than being a value in itself. In other words, during a Low scenario, £500/$900 could buy me an ounce of gold or 2,000 cans of tinned beans. Those cans of beans will keep my family alive for a year, but what good will the gold do us? If the time comes when survival is of primary interest, you may not be able to trade your ounce of gold for 2,000 cans of beans. You may not even be able to trade it for a single can. The value of anything is simply what you can trade for it, and when it comes down to a choice between a lovely metal and a filling meal, you can be assured that most of us will opt for the latter.

How the pandemic can turn the property bubble into a lead balloon

Land and property investment is a very interesting case. The valuations of real property in most developed countries have increased well above the reach of the average worker in the past couple of decades. The unreasonable and unprecedented spike in property prices has created a new caste system. The Brahmins already own property and can live lavishly just by remortgaging their ever-increasing asset, and the Untouchables are destined to rent for eternity, as the prospect of ever coming up with a down payment or qualifying for a mortgage payment equal or greater than their entire monthly salary is nothing but a vague dream.

The prices of property almost everywhere have skyrocketed, but even in this booming worldwide market, there are still absolutely staggering differences in pricing for essentially the same house, simply based on geography. Let's consider two houses, both essentially similar, and listed for sale in the summer of 2005. Four bedrooms, two bathrooms, about 186 square metres on a reasonable lot with a two-car garage, and built in the 20th century. They are both in pleasant, calm, leafy suburban neighbourhoods in English-speaking, stable, peaceful countries. They contain about the same fixtures and appliances. They are almost identical in every way. The difference is that house number one is in Amersham, Bucks, England and house number two is in Swift Current, Saskatchewan, Canada. Through most of the year they have a similar climate, although Saskatchewan does experience a rather rigid winter. But the real difference is in the price. House Number One is on the market at £599,000/$1,078,200. House Number Two is also for sale, but for close to £40,000/$72,000. How one house can cost fifteen times more than the other is not just an illustration of the tired old estate agent chestnut 'location, location, location', but a way to comprehend what the value of a house really is. The cost of the building materials, labour, etc that went into the Saskatchewan house doesn't vary too much from the English house. The former is brick over stud construction and the latter brick over block but that doesn't affect the cost to any great degree. The only real difference in the valuation is that Amersham is believed to be a more desirable place to live than Swift Current. Now, I've been to both places, and I can assure you that as long as you don't go to Swift Current in January, it is a wonderful town. Personally, I'd pick it over Amersham. But while you can jump on the Tube in Amersham and be in Leicester Square in an hour, the only place you can be in an hour from Swift Current is right smack in the middle of nowhere.

But what if the middle of nowhere became more attractive than Leicester Square? What if the charms of a magnificent metropolis such as London suddenly turned into nightmares? What if people shunned places such as Leicester Square for its teeming masses of infectious flu victims and wanted to be isolated and safe? Then the house in Swift Current might be worth more than the one in Amersham.

You can take this relative economy one step further. I found a not-luxurious but perfectly serviceable two bedroom house on a large lot not far from Swift Current selling for £1,800/$3,240. That wouldn't even buy you one square metre of the Amersham house and is far less than its annual council tax. And if you can't handle chilly winters, you may find similar values in small out-of-the-way towns in Western Australia or the Northern Territory that might be better suited to you.

Property values are illusory at best. It is all part hype, part expectation, and part delusion. You charge what the market will bear because everyone else around you is. The house itself is really only worth the cost of the materials and labour that turned the previously empty lot into a residence.

This is a lesson that is very important to learn when considering property investment in a global crisis such as a pandemic. The proximity to lots of exciting people is exactly what you might not want. And as soon as the people around you start thinking in the same way, they might want to get away from you and the people near you as well. That's when the pendulum can shift. 'Totally isolated at the end of a 32-km dirt road' might become the selling point that 'easy access to the city' is today.

This logic also extends to another popular investment in many countries around the world, a Real Estate Investment Trust (REIT), which is a wide-spectrum property investment portfolio traded on the stock market. A REIT is a company set up primarily to own and manage investment properties. It's basically a way to buy shares in a variety of properties. If those properties are in areas where the prices are going up, then the value of each share of the REIT goes up. REITs have seemed to be fuelled by perpetual-motion machines, as they have been going up and up and up since they were introduced. That is because their performance is tied into the insane spiral of house pricing that has only recently begun to abate. However, in the pandemic age, it might be wise to seek out a REIT that invests in more rural and secluded properties as those may very well be the ones that at least maintain their current real values.

The lesson is to not be hypnotised by high property values. The justification for asking those prices can swiftly dissipate and the entire pattern of real estate valuation can be tipped upside down. All it takes is one little 0.1-micron virus.

Sector by sector forecast of stock market performance through a pandemic

We've glanced at various investments and how they might fare in a pandemic era. However, not all investments are bound to have negative yields through a pandemic. Let's take a look at a possible forecast by sector along with prospect of share prices immediately post-pandemic in the Low and Medium Severity scenarios:

Beat the Flu

Type of Share	Low Severity scenario	Medium Severity scenario
Aerospace and Defence	The Aerospace component would be affected by absenteeism but Defence will likely strengthen on the call for greater security at border points and general international xenophobia. **Prospect: Aerospace – Down 20%; Defence – Up 15%**	The Aerospace industry will come to a screeching halt, but Defence will skyrocket. The prospect of entire continents being sealed off to all comers will create a huge demand for all sorts of security and military equipment with enormous price tags. **Prospect: Aerospace – Down 70%; Defence – Up 30%**
Automobiles	Walloped by factory- and sales-floor absenteeism and by ordinary people staying home, this will be one of the hardest-hit sectors. When people are afraid to go outside is not the time they will be shopping for new cars. **Prospect: Down 30%**	Absenteeism will all but shut down the factories and there won't be much point in producing cars as nobody will be buying. Many international, storied marques will disappear forever. Commercial vehicles will not be hit as hard as private cars. **Prospect: Down 60%**
Banks	A surprisingly vulnerable sector. Their astronomical profits will crash down to earth as property values deflate. Just as people won't rate buying a new car as a priority, they won't be buying a new house or factory either. **Prospect: Down 25%**	This sector's vulnerability will be further exposed by the collapse in Residential and Commercial Property values and the plummeting stock market. Too many banks will be over-stretched and will disappear in a flurry of bad debts and inability to dispose of repossessed assets. **Prospect: Down 75%**
Beverages	Should stay somewhat untouched, and shop alcohol sales may even rise at the expense of pub profits. It's not a great idea to spend the night drinking in a crowded pub or bar, but the overall situation may call for belting down more than the usual back at home. **Prospect: Up 5%**	If anything is going to drive people to drink, a pandemic is it. As the local dries up, the home will be awash in booze. Consumption could increase by 50% but it will all be off-licence sales. Even though transport is in shambles, people will always find some way to get alcohol. Companies that can deliver liquor to the home will boom. **Prospect: Up 20%**

Surviving the Pandemic Financially

Type of Share	Low Severity scenario	Medium Severity scenario
Chemicals	Will be hit by the general economic malaise and absenteeism resulting in lower productivity. Demand will be down for most of this sector as retail and manufacturing slow down. **Prospect: Down 20%**	The only chemical manufacturers to benefit will be the ones producing materials that go into pharmaceuticals, alternative medicines, food preservation and embalming. All other aspects of this sector will swiftly crumble. **Prospect: Down 60%**
Construction and Building Materials	In this extremely labour-intensive industry where most of the work is carried out outdoors, you can expect some of the highest absentee rates of any sector. New construction will slow to a crawl as property deflation takes hold. **Prospect: Down 25%**	The only construction going on will likely be with salvaged materials by people setting up shelters in rural areas away from the mass deaths in the cities. The trade as it currently exists may virtually vanish not to return for many years. **Prospect: Down 90%**
Distributors	It depends what they are distributing. Higher end discretionary products will tank. Food and staple necessities will benefit significantly. The bottom-line question in this sector along with many others is: do people really need that product? If yes, the company will be a winner. If not, a loser. **Prospect: Discretionary Distributors – Down 30%; Necessity Distributors – Up 15%**	Again, it depends what they are distributing. Higher-end discretionary products will simply cease to exist. Food and staple necessities will be the only products that sell. However, problems with the distribution matrix and the inability to physically get the products to the buyers will bring the entire sector down. **Prospect: Discretionary Distributors – Down 90%; Necessity Distributors – Down 25%**
Diversified Industrials	Diminished demand and factory-floor absenteeism will affect this sector profoundly. Some industrials will flourish, especially in the domestic consumable, sanitation and alternative energy areas, but most will suffer. **Prospect: Overall Down 15%**	Domestic consumables, sanitation and alternative energy providers will survive, but most will simply shut down. The impossibility of getting staff to the factories, combined with disappearing demand for anything but the barest necessities will ravage this sector. **Prospect: Down 70%**

Beat the Flu

Type of Share	Low Severity scenario	Medium Severity scenario
Electricity	A clear winner. The pandemic and the resultant skewing of overall energy demand from transportation to electricity will allow as a convenient excuse for price-gouging as rates will go up due to the emergency situation. People switching to telecommuting will drive electric demand up as well. **Prospect: Up 30%**	Absenteeism will create a vicious chain reaction in lowering electricity supply at the time when the demand is the highest in history. Generating plants will have to shut down due to lack of staff to operate and maintain the equipment. Blackouts will be a common daily occurrence. Raising prices will not help as the blackouts will cut the kilowatt-per-house level down by half or more. **Prospect: Down 40%**
Electronics and Electrical	When half your household is home with a potentially lethal flu is not the time you think of going electronics shopping. This sector will be hit as hard as the rest of discretionary retail. **Prospect: Down 20%**	This sector will follow electricity into the rubbish heap. No point having electrical appliances when there is no electricity flowing through the mains. Generators may boom, but the problem of getting the fuel to run them may stifle that demand as well. **Prospect: Down 80%**
Engineering	The stock market drop will savage Engineering and Research and Development. New product and project developments will be cancelled or delayed as the capital of the companies who pay for it dries up. **Prospect: Down 30%**	Engineering and Research and Development for all intents and purposes will cease to exist as new projects and product development are irrevocably cancelled due to lack of funds and staffing. It may not return to any health whatsoever for at least five years. **Prospect: Down 95%**
Food Processing	All agricultural-related companies will do well as increased transportation costs act as a good excuse for price-raising. People will be stocking up on shelf-stable food products, thus this sector can strengthen if it can overcome its absenteeism problems. **Prospect: Up 15%**	Again, absenteeism and transportation impossibilities will hit this sector hard. Even though the demand for food will be high, the bottlenecks will crush this industry. Without any other choices, people will turn to growing their own food or even scavenging. **Prospect: Down 50%**

Surviving the Pandemic Financially

Type of Share	Low Severity scenario	Medium Severity scenario
Football Clubs	There has already been talk of the government cancelling or curtailing entire sporting seasons. The thought of spending a cold rainy evening out in a stadium with 50,000 strangers is not comforting during a pandemic. There will be a staggering dip, but this sector will likely rebound quickly. **Prospect: Down 25%, but returning to normal within six months**	As football-mad as many people may be, sporting events will be indefinitely cancelled as prime contagion opportunities. It will be several years before they return in any organised fashion and in the meantime the leagues will likely be disbanded. **Prospect: Zero**
Gas Distribution	Like Electricity, this sector is a gold standard winner. Rising rates, driven by panic and higher household usage, will push profitability into previously uncharted territory. **Prospect: Up 30%**	This sector will suffer the same paradoxical problems as Electricity. Demand at an all-time high but profound inability to deliver. Unlike electricity, however, gas distribution will have an additional problem. Absenteeism in the maintenance staff will cause several large and damaging explosions which may end up shutting down the network altogether. **Prospect: Down 75%**
Health and Pharmaceuticals	There are different subsectors in Health and each will perform differently. Folk remedies, alternative medicine and allopathic flu relief will skyrocket, as will hospital consumables. Fitness and related products will suffer as people stay home. Other components of this sector should flatline. **Prospect: Flu-related – Up 35%; Non-flu related – Down 5%**	No bright stars here, at least not any more. By now, the majority of the public has realised that there is nothing that can be taken to alleviate flu symptoms or stem the mortality rate. This sector collapses all for hospital consumables. **Prospect: Down 70%**

Type of Share	Low Severity scenario	Medium Severity scenario
Household	Another split situation. Any company that has anything to do with stocking and storing of food, water, and other household necessities will benefit from people stripping the shelves at their local stores. Shortages will drive prices way up. Household luxuries and anything that is strictly non-necessary will drop. **Prospect: Necessities – Up 25%; Discretionary – Down 10%**	By this time the shelves are bare and the stores that were in the retail channel have closed, so this sector is ruined. Transportation and absenteeism problems choke off what little production there was. **Prospect: Down 80%**
Information Technology Hardware	Corporate demand will dry up but household demand will take off as more people set themselves up to tele-commute and cocoon in their homes. Home PCs will be upgraded to facilitate working at home. Domestic installation and repair companies will be swamped. **Prospect: Corporate – Down – 25%; Domestic – Up 30%**	Corporate demand is gone and the problem of receiving a steady electricity supply kills off household demand as well. There will still be a market for repairing computers damaged by the frequent voltage spikes of the unreliable electric supply, but it will mostly be from used and scavenged parts. **Prospect: Down 70%**
Insurance	This industry will be hit hard through cancelled vehicle policies and big pay-offs on life insurance. It will try to raise its premiums but find significant public resistance. Insurance is one of the big losers. **Prospect: Down 40%**	Most insurers will be in massive default by this time. Life insurance policies will be paid out at a few percentage of the policy values at first and then not at all. Loss of liquidity will shut down most insurers, including some of the biggest names in the industry. **Prospect: Down 90%**
Internet	As clear a winner as Electricity or Gas. People will spend much more time at home and will want to communicate and surf the	Another case of too much demand and inability to supply. Electricity outages will strangle internet access as too many users

Type of Share	Low Severity scenario	Medium Severity scenario
	net at unheard-of levels. Much of their buying will shift to online retailers creating a boom for home-delivery companies. ISPs would be well advised to invest in that new server farm today. **Prospect: Up 30%** **Low Severity scenario**	logging on at the same time after blackouts will cause entire sections of the web to collapse. Absenteeism will affect ISP's ability to keep their servers running and the whole situation will escalate into a major disaster. **Prospect: Down 75%**
Investment Trusts	They will suffer the same doldrums as the rest of the market and the general direction is down. The few astute fund managers who shift their portfolios towards the few sectors that are due to rise will be heralded as prophetic geniuses. The rest will be massacred. **Prospect: Down 25%**	As goes the market, so go the trusts, but even more so. Investment will not be the first priority in most people's minds, survival will be. **Prospect: Zero**
Leisure	A bad time to be in this industry. Holiday packagers, restaurants, pubs and hotels during a pandemic will be hit hard by absenteeism and vanishing demand. They all deal in providing access to crowded areas, which is exactly where you don't want to be in a pandemic. **Prospect: Down 35%**	Holiday packagers, restaurants and pubs will be sealed up and forgotten. Hotels will continue to operate, but only as makeshift hospitals and morgues. Rural hotels will be taken over by force by refugees from the contagion pits of the cities. **Prospect: Down 85%**
Media	Hollywood studios will delay releases and broadcast networks will see their advertising revenue plummet. DVD sales and rentals will suffer significantly but pay-for-view will show huge gains. Furthermore, all of the kids stuck at home may boost video-game sales and news networks will do well as they always do in international crises. **Prospect: Down 20%**	The closure of cinemas and irregular electricity supplies to the home will flatten this sector. People will rush to watch television when the electricity flows, but there will be much time when it does not. Entertainment programming will effectively disappear, replaced by bulletins from skeleton news crews. **Prospect: Down 70%**

Type of Share	Low Severity scenario	Medium Severity scenario
Mining	Absenteeism combined with industrial slowdown will significantly damage this sector. Coal mining may find a second wind due to householders seeking alternative energy sources, but overall, this is a vulnerable group. **Prospect: Down 25%**	For now, it will shut down, but it may return as a shadow of its former self post-pandemic. **Prospect: Down 90%**
Oil and Petrol	The shift from transportation demand to household demand will be jarring but it should keep this industry fairly healthy. The market for petrol will be halved or less, but diesel for transportation of goods and agriculture will stay strong. Petrol will benefit from the higher rates the distributors will charge. **Prospect: Up 10%**	Transportation fuel demand has all but disappeared as the international transport network creaks to a halt. There will be a high demand for household and heating fuels, but transportation bottlenecks will make it impossible to get the supply to markets. **Prospect: Down 60%**
Personal Care and Household Products	Anything that is a luxury is a goner. Cosmetics, perfumes and other products to prepare individuals for social contact will suffer significant losses. Personal hygiene and kitchen necessities will see increased demand. **Prospect: Down 20%**	Another effective shutdown due to absenteeism, transportation impossibilities and a vanishing distribution matrix. **Prospect: Down 80%**
Real Estate	Residential and Commercial property values will be in freefall. Supply will far outstrip the weak to non-existent demand. Urban properties will be hard hit, while there will be a boom in isolated country properties as those who can afford it look seriously at abandoning the teeming, contagious cities. The industrial slowdown and factory closings will collapse commercial prices. **Prospect: Down 40%**	Property values? What property values? City property will be next to worthless as contagion increases and law and order breaks down. Some rural properties, especially the larger and more isolated ones, may actually increase in value, but there will be a serious shortage of cash to purchase any of them. Commercial property will be overrun by squatters and vandals. **Prospect: Down 75%**

Surviving the Pandemic Financially

Type of Share	Low Severity scenario	Medium Severity scenario
Retailers	Most retailers sell impulse and discretionary items and they will see their sales floors empty. The low-paid store staff will also fail to show up and the absentee rate may be the highest of any sector. When you factor in the huge shift to online purchasing from people who are afraid to leave their houses, the outlook is very bleak for all retailers not in the market of necessary staple products. **Prospect: Down 35%**	Retail is gone. It will make a comeback but will likely never again see current levels. The high street as we know it won't be seen soon, if ever. **Prospect: Down 85%**
Software	The pandemic may be the best promoter of electronic entertainment and activities. Software that facilitates online commerce and leisure will be well positioned. Online-downloaded software will have the significant edge over programs on CD or DVD that must be purchased in a store. **Prospect: Up 25%**	This sector will follow the rest of IT. Everyone wants to use it, but they can't because there is too little electricity generated. **Prospect: Down 75%**
Speciality	Wipeout. Most of this sector falls specifically into the discretionary portion of the product spectrum and will be the first to fall. Some major global brands will merge or disappear altogether. **Prospect: Down 35%**	You've got to be kidding! **Prospect: Zero**
Steel and Metals	Manufacturing and construction down and thus this sector will follow. With no bright spots to be able to identify and absenteeism at an all-time high, some big names in this sector will be bankrupt. **Prospect: Down 25%**	Gone the way of mining, but it will return several years in the future. **Prospect: Down 90%**

Type of Share	Low Severity scenario	Medium Severity scenario
Telecommunications Services	The shift to a home-based economy will boost telecom stocks to new highs, although not to the dizzying heights of internet companies. Landlines will make a comeback at the expense of mobile phones as people find themselves at home much longer than usual. **Prospect: Up 15%**	Landline telecom is as reliant on electric supply as any other industry, so the blackouts will be compounded by absenteeism and inability to service and maintain the networks. Significant degradation of the physical infrastructure will mean that landlines may never return and be replaced by a new generation of wireless telecom that can handle large amounts of data for internet usage, but that will be several years in the future. **Prospect: Down 75%**
Tobacco	Just like alcoholic beverages will benefit from the pandemic, so will tobacco, as worries and increased time at home will boost consumption. Black-market distribution will take up much of the increase in high-tax countries. **Prospect: Up 15%**	The impossibility of getting tobacco from the growing areas to the developed countries will stifle this industry. Demand will be overwhelming, a pack of cigarettes will cost more than a week's groceries, but soon there will be no more to go around. Forced to quit by non-existent supplies, many smokers will not return when supplies do. **Prospect: Down 50%**
Transport	All aspects of this sector will suffer and lower petrol prices will not help much. All forms of people transport will suffer as passenger numbers drop to unheard-of levels. Home delivery companies and food transporters are the only shining stars in this sullied firmament. **Prospect: Down 30%**	The other triggering point for the economic meltdown next to electricity. Transport companies cannot provide services as they lack the staff, there is plenty of fuel but it can't be distributed, and the whole situation spirals into disaster. **Prospect: Down 60%**

High Severity

That brings us to the High Severity scenario. I stated that this was the apocalyptic option and truly it is. At this level of worldwide impact, all bets are off.

Stock markets would effectively cease to operate and this would have a disastrous effect on the world economies. With investments wiped out, cash could take a predominant position, but the unwise knee-jerk reactions of some politicians could cause Weimar Republic-style hyperinflation, wiping out its value and sparking a barter economy. Even precious metals could suffer as people would find little practical use for gold. Bonds would be useless paper. The Bond Markets as we know them would cease to exist with barter becoming the operative economic model. Bonds are built on trust in the future and this would be a very rare commodity in a pandemic economy. The global panic would delay the return to a stable Bond Market for at least a full generation.

Social upheaval is certain to follow the inability of governments to provide health care and vaccines to the vast majority of their populations. Imagine that there is only enough antiviral or vaccine for 5 per cent of your national population and it's reserved only for government and health essential personnel. Break-ins and armed robberies in hospitals and pharmacies to get these drugs would be the order of the day. As fatalities mounted, mass hysteria could set in, with people willing to do literally anything to secure food and supplies. A survival-at-all-costs mentality could become pervasive. Police and military would be swamped by this unrest, as well as their own internal casualties due to flu and clashes with a very violent citizenry.

There are no real hedges in this eventuality, whether financial or social, and the survivalist's credo that the only things of real value are 'food, water and ammunition' could actually come to pass.

There is no point analysing this option sector by sector. After the pandemic claims 500 million or more people, civilisation will not return to the Stone Age, but it might be pretty close. We can rest assured that there will be a very different world on the other side of a pandemic this pervasive.

Science will be shunned as it offered no hope when humanity needed it most. The prospect of basing a world economy on a bubble of credit and ever-higher, but essentially irrational, expectations will never return. Survival issues will be much closer to the forefront of Western nations, which previously concerned themselves with more esoteric and abstract pursuits. The breakdown of law and order will see some communities band together and operate their own vigilante, Wild-West justice. Atrocities now limited to warring tribes in Central Africa will become commonplace.

The elimination of the financial system may spur a new Golden Age or we may just descend into savagery. No one can know. Does humanity have within it the ability to build a new, better, fairer and truly utopian system on the ashes of the deceased world, or will we just return to a Dark Age feudalism where we band together only for self-preservation from the savages outside the walls?

The world of 1918 was very different to today's. In almost a century we have seen the evolution of a very different human paradigm where Western civilisation has become fully dependent on technology and its trappings. As to whether this dependence can be reversed to return to self-reliance and manual labour is questionable, especially in light of having to bury nearly one out of every ten of us. This world cannot absorb in a year a dozen times the casualties that it has taken HIV to accumulate in more than a quarter-century. Something has to break. This pandemic will strike at the core of this very civilisation, in the heart of its crowded cities where H5N1 will spread between us as a swift, horrible, invisible killer. I can only hope that in this scenario, humanity will finally distinguish itself as the noble animal we can be.

CHAPTER 13

Going the Extra Mile to Stay Safe

How you can prepare for these Low, Medium and High Severity scenarios

It is well worth repeating what I stated in an earlier chapter: *Keep in mind that these worst possible case scenarios have a very tiny percentage possibility of ever occurring. This pandemic may never come. Don't worry yourself into an early grave over the prospect.*

However, you're reading this book because you have seen the media reports about this stealthy killer coming our way and you want to know more about it. If at the end of this book you have been sufficiently convinced that this is serious and it's real, then you will take some measure of precaution to help keep yourself and your loved ones safe from this modern plague. Some may go overboard, but most of you will just take a tip here and there and apply them at your judgement. Maybe some will walk around with respirators. Hopefully more will wash their hands carefully. All of those suggestions are good ones and will certainly help keep you free from the virus. Note that I wrote 'help' keep you free from the virus. These precautions, as good as they may be, cannot guarantee that you will not get infected with H5N1.

Going the Extra Mile to Stay Safe

Remember: none of this may happen. This could all just be for nothing. H5N1 could simply engage in antigenic shift with some strange virus and go off on an evolutionary vector that does not cross the path of *Homo sapiens*. In that case, we can all merrily go about our business and won't have to prepare for such a vicious global cull of humanity – from H5N1 anyway.

However, there are many of us that believe that it will happen, and indeed it's right around the corner. This is not just some mad cult of crazies fixing the date and time of Armageddon and then when that date passes, setting up another one in the future. We can track the explosion of H5N1 from its origins in Eastern Asia to many other countries. We can see how it progressed, how it infected, how it killed. At every step along the way there were always the naysayers who stated that, yes it's gone this far but it won't go any further. And at every step along the way they were wrong.

You shouldn't consider yourself (or me for that matter) an apocalyptic nutcase for preparing for this eventuality. The people who have reasonable precautions ready will be far better equipped to survive and thrive through the pandemic. If the pandemic never happens, then little is lost anyway. You can always sell off or use your food stock and supplies.

That brings us down to the critical question: if you are to believe that one of the three severity scenarios will indeed unfold, what can you do, in hard and fast terms right now, to take precautions for your family?

Let's analyse the steps that you can take today to prepare for these three scenarios. I'll jump ahead a bit and advise you that the effective, practical preparations for the High Severity scenario are next to nothing. The only truly effective precautions are so Draconian that most people simply cannot conceive of implementing any of them. I'm listing them anyway but I doubt whether even I will be prepared to this degree. But I am preparing for the Low and to a certain degree even the Medium scenarios. You can bet that if the pandemic arrives, I'll be as ready as I can be for it!

The Low Severity scenario

You can stock up on Sharp Plasmaclusters and N-100 masks and 55-gallon drums of bleach and Virkon S and still will not be able to guarantee that H5N1 will not find its way into your system. Inhalation and ingestion of a microscopic virus is far too easy in a pandemic situation. The virus could be anywhere. Anyone you pass on the street may be infected and may not even know that they are contagious yet. Absolute safety is effectively unattainable.

The only 100 per cent guaranteed way to not catch H5N1 is not to be in contact with anyone or anything that has the virus. It seems like a very simple precaution, but it is one that most people simply cannot imagine. Let's assume that you are going to sit the pandemic out at your home and that, of course, it's a Low Severity scenario. There are a mind-boggling array of preparations you need to take. Scrimp or cut out any one of them and you may be asking for serious trouble down the road.

The first consideration is: where? Naturally, we would all say at home. That may not be as simple as you might first think. If you are living in a fully-detached home then you can skip this part. But most people live in semi-detached, terrace houses, flats or apartment buildings. That's where it becomes more complicated.

We have to consider airflow. Does your residence share air vents with any other nearby apartment or house? Many apartments with forced air heating have all the units interconnected through the ventilation system. That is big trouble, since you can stay in your unit throughout the entire pandemic but if you're breathing in the air that has just circulated throughout the entire building you might as well go to work in a crowded office.

You need to filter the air that comes into your environment and the best way to do that is with vent filters. Make sure that you pick a type that has the smallest mesh, measured in microns, that you can find. Also ensure that the vent filter fits snugly in the opening and is taped securely all the way around to keep air from sneaking in. Even the return air vents that take air out of your apartment need to be filtered. Forced air HVAC turns itself on and off as required, thus the return air vent can actually bring air into your area when the system shuts down.

If you're feeling particularly wealthy, try placing a Sharp Plasmacluster in front of each and every air vent. It's an expensive option and will only work if the electricity isn't turned off, but it will significantly lower the levels of airborne H5N1 in your apartment.

However, filtering the vents is not going to give you the absolute safety you're seeking. If you live in a place like this, the best thing you can do is find somewhere else to sit out the pandemic. This is of course a minority solution. It will be well-nigh impractical for the majority of urban dwellers to find a nice place in the isolated country to wait out the pandemic. Furthermore, unless you are quick off the mark, you will find that all the other urban dwellers that had the same idea have beaten you to it. The worst thing that can happen in this residential transferring process is that you are left homeless with nowhere to stay in city or country. Also keep in mind that all of this is strictly speculative since, depending on the progress of the pandemic, the government may quarantine major towns and cities. The press have already forecast martial law and mass quarantines, and in October 2005 President Bush made a statement that any part of the United States where H5N1 breaks out could face a military-enforced quarantine.

If you are seeking an alternative and more virus-secure residence, detached houses are not just best, they are the only way to go. And if the house is on a very large lot or acreage, better still. Some older country houses sit on very large lots but the house is squished in just inches from the road. That is useless. You want a house that is completely isolated from its neighbours with as much distance from any other building as you can achieve.

This may be too optimal but if you could find one with a clean stream on the property that comes directly down from the hills and nowhere near a town and has been lab tested to be safe to drink, that would help immensely in taking care of your single biggest requirement: water.

Keep in mind that we are not discussing moving permanently. In the Low Severity scenario, we are only looking for a place to spend a few months, possibly as little as two and maybe as many as four or five. Then the pandemic will abate and it will all be over.

The key is to be aware of when the pandemic is coming. You don't want to leave your home prematurely but you also don't want to wait until it's too late. There is no point becoming infected with H5N1 in the city and then moving out to the country taking your virus with you to infect the rural residents. This is a delicate balancing act that can best be performed with information. Keep an eye on the news, check the internet and be ready to move quickly when it's announced that H5N1 is here and people are starting to get sick. I'd use the proximity radius as a rule of thumb. When reports show human-to-human infective transmission about 500 km from you, it's time to hit the road. Not next week, but today. And this is assuming that you already have your location fully stocked with everything you need. By this time it will be too late to go shopping for the huge amount of supplies you will need.

Make sure that your vehicle is always filled to the brim with fuel and in good mechanical condition. The last thing you need is to get stuck on the way to your shelter house.

There are two somewhat reasonable options. The first and cheapest one is to locate some good friends or family that have a suitable country house and are equally concerned about the pandemic and pay them to move in with them. In most cases the payment will be minimal and you can probably bring extra supplies for them as your rent. It's important that these people are as serious as you about waiting out the pandemic and taking all possible precautions. It's not going to help if you are well sheltered in the country and one of them decides that they have to go into town to buy chocolates.

To keep complete control over the residential situation, the best option is to rent a country house. You will actually be surprised how many country homes are available for rent in rural areas, especially in the off-peak season. For a reasonable two-bedroom detached house with land around it you're likely to pay less than you would for a one-bedroom small apartment in a city. A small price to pay for this level of safety. If you're getting your own place make sure that you have at least one and preferably several more like-minded people to come with you. Not only can you share the expenses, but if you share your time with people whose company you enjoy, the time may well pass much more quickly. Most importantly, other people can help you if you fall ill.

Make sure that you pay the landlord in advance for the entire period you expect to stay in the house. The last thing you need is for him and his viruses to come over and try and collect rent. If you have a UV portable flashlight, use it to decontaminate all your post. If you don't have one, stop the mail and have it held at the post office so that the postman won't come over. Seal the mail slot and if anyone drops anything by outside your door, leave it there.

If you have found a location, it's time to stock it. You would actually be astonished at how much you need. Let's assume that you are planning for four months of isolation. The mountain of food for this period of time is going to be gargantuan. Find a bulk store that will give you a volume discount, or call around to find food wholesalers that will cut you a deal. Don't worry too much about having the best quality or your favourite foods. Maybe you won't have much lobster and lots of tinned beans, but you can treat yourself once the pandemic has subsided.

It's important to plan nutritionally balanced meals featuring reasonable levels of protein, carbohydrates and fat that are calorie controlled to compensate for your lower activity level. You should not require more than 1,800 calories (kilocalories, of course) a day for men and 1,500 for women. Most of the time you are going to be sitting around and won't be burning up those calories. Canned, jarred and dried food is best. Don't stock anything that won't last four months without refrigeration, so foodstuffs like strawberries and fresh meats are out. There are lots of canned meats, vegetables and fruits available and various and various dried beef, kippers and other meats and fishes that are delicious and packed with nutrition. Rice, cereals and pastas are lifesavers. Don't even bother with refrigerated foods and forget frozen foods, as if the electricity supply fails for a day you've wasted it all. Try to avoid alcohol and narcotics. You will need your sobriety for the challenges ahead.

For each person you will need to take along 360 meals. That is a lot of food! Three meals a day for four months. Forget large cooked breakfasts. You can settle for muesli and long-life milk. Eat simply and wholesomely. Try to create menus that don't require cooking, or if they do, can be simply prepared in a single pot. Fuel for cooking may become an issue. Plan out each and every one of those meals so that you have absolutely everything you need. You won't be able to just run to the corner store for some ketchup.

Water is the single biggest problem you'll have. If you are lucky enough to have found a house with a stream nearby you can always have a fresh supply. You'll have to boil every drop first, even for bathing, but if cooking fuel is not an issue that is by far the best way to get your water. If you don't have this optimal situation, then you need to store your own water. You cannot rely on the utilities staying on. There may be no water, gas or electricity for some or all of the time you are battened down. Be ready.

You will have to allow for about 12 litres of water per person per day. And that is just for drinking, cooking and sponging yourself down. No baths, showers or toilet flushing. That is a huge amount of water over four months.

Over this period, each person will need 1,362 litres of water, which will take up 1.36 cubic metres. That is a lot of space. It's like a column of water 61 centimetres wide, 91 centimetres deep and all the way from the floor to the ceiling. If you are planning for six people to last out the pandemic you will need enough water to fill a small bedroom right up to chest level.

Your food storage space requirements will likely equal your water. You are going to need a lot of space to store your supplies, so make sure that you are prepared for that.

Other indispensable items are lots of basic, sturdy clothes, cold and rain gear, several good torches, lots of fresh batteries, candles, stay-dry matches, tools, razors, cutlery, dishes, cups, pots, toilet paper, painkillers, a sewing kit, playing cards, games, books and best of all washing-up liquid. You can use it for every washing purpose from the one intended all the way to laundry and shampoo. Of course have at least a gallon of thin bleach per person per week with you, and make sure you have a comprehensive first-aid kit. Make sure that at least two of the people with you are trained in first aid. Fuel is critical. Don't count on the electricity or the gas staying on. If you are in a wooded area have a good axe handy and use it carefully.

A readily available wind-up radio is priceless. Keep abreast of news developments. Don't leave until the news announces that the pandemic has completely passed. As long as the ISPs stay in function, broadband is a necessity to keep in touch with the outside world. It's also worth remembering to take plenty of books and board games to pass the time. You don't want boredom making you take risks, such as venturing outside.

Of course you need cash and lots of it. Empty your bank account and savings and turn it all into lower denomination banknotes that are easy to use for smaller purchases. Keep lots of cash with you in a very safe place at all times, as the whole idea is that you are not going to be able to get to a bank machine or anywhere else people are. Besides, your bank may fail during the pandemic and your cash is safer with you than in some failed bank's computer memory.

This is only a brief summary, as there is lots more information that you can garner from conventional survivalist books and websites. Keep in mind that you are planning for complete isolation. You don't want to go out hunting or fishing as that could be a vector for the virus right into your otherwise safe house. Just because it's bird flu doesn't mean only people and birds have it. It could have undergone antigenic shifting and thus be present in virtually any other mammal, reptile or even fish. The only reason you want to go outside is to fetch water. If you do decide to get some air, don't sit or lie down on anything and leave a special set of shoes outside, in case you walk on H5N1 infected bird droppings. And if anyone comes to the door, don't open it and simply shoo them away.

Keep in mind that these tactics may only delay the inevitable. When the 1918 virus spread from Kansas to each one of the 48 contiguous United States, even without the benefit of jet travel, it swiftly reached the most isolated regions. The reality is that there may be virtually no habitable place on earth that can be termed completely safe.

Now if saving or sustaining your business is one of your top priorities you will need to implement a pandemic-ready plan for your business. This is a multiple-step process. The first step is to ensure the safety and continuity of your workforce. Issue respirators, goggles and rubber gloves and make sure that they use them. Train them in handwashing and hygiene procedures. Discourage them from social contact outside of work. Secure your customer contact areas so that the only face-to-face contact with your clients occurs through hermetically sealed glass and intercoms. Ensure that you have adequate backup supplies, consumables and 'off the grid' energy capability. Overstock yourself to the limit and beyond, regardless of how you have to pay or not pay for it. When your competition has empty shelves you will be swarmed with customers.

Don't leave your capital in the bank. Bury boxes full of cash under your house if you have to, but don't trust any electronic systems with your business' lifeblood. Safeguard your data and records. Make a full backup of absolutely everything on separate hard drives and take them out of the building. Keep them safe at home, never in a bank safety deposit box. Remember, your bank might not be around in a few months. Stop accepting credit, debit cards and cheques. You may not get the money.

If you're in a rarefied upper-echelon business, such as Rolex or Ferrari sales, consider switching to staples for the duration of the pandemic. Keep in mind that there will be precious little demand for £15,000/$27,000 wristwatches but overwhelming demand for Pot Noodles. If you are one of those businesspeople who would sell bottled water for $100 in flooded New Orleans and can bear the foray into repugnant, macabre opportunism, these items should be in incredible demand: air filters and purifiers, alcohol hand sanitisers, antiviral and vaccine (if you can get it), batteries, bleach, bottled water, camp stoves, candles, dried, canned and jarred food, electric generators, first aid kits, folk flu remedies (regardless of efficacy), fuel of any kind, funeral and morgue supplies, goggles, heat pads, hydrogen peroxide, inhalers, respirators, rubber gloves, rubbing alcohol, stay-dry matches, survivalist and camping gear, water filters and purifiers, and wind-up radios.

However, if you have spare funds I very much urge you to take it upon yourself to distribute as much of this stock as possible where needed for free. You will get good media coverage, and people will remember your company's good will when the pandemic is over.

The Medium Severity scenario

This is a far more severe scenario than the Low Severity. While during that scenario we were expecting that the electricity and gas may go out, now we are counting on it. We also didn't consider personal safety during the Low scenario, but now we must.

During a Medium Severity scenario the choice of location becomes more critical. The preferred places are extremely isolated, preferably on their own dirt road. You can cut down a tree and let it fall across the entrance to the road to discourage wanderers.

Note that a Medium scenario can last six to eight months, so you can just take all the supplies that were mentioned for the Low Severity scenario and double the quantities. Furthermore, water supplies cannot be trusted, so having all your own water is obligatory. The small bedroom filled with water to chest level will now have to be right up to the ceiling. The same with the food storage. It is an enormous amount of stuff.

You will definitely need fuel for cooking and staying warm. I don't advise storing that much liquid fuel, as it is far too much of a fire risk. You will have to ensure that there is plenty of dry or dryable hardwood in the immediate area and that you can get to it. When you go out, make sure you have your respirator, goggles and rubber gloves on at all times.

The seriousness of the people with you is critical as well. Six to eight months is an astounding amount of time to be spent cooped up with difficult or cranky people. You will all have to be dedicated to your ongoing safety and be able to get along over the long haul.

Ensure that all the bills for the house and anything else you can think of are paid well in advance so no one will have reason to come over. Think of everything to have your location just disappear from public perception.

Now comes the tough part, and the one where I'll be in disagreement with most of my readers. I'm sorry, but you will need to take whatever steps necessary to protect yourself and your loved ones. A Medium scenario can escalate to a High pandemic very quickly and, in that case, law and order may disappear within days. If a group of raiders want your stash the only thing between them and your survival may be your courage and how well prepared you are.

A Medium Severity pandemic will be far harder for your business to survive than the Low scenario where you could conceivably come out ahead. You should stop thinking about how to profit. Right now you just want your business to survive in more or less one piece.

Again, your personnel is key. Clear out some warehouse or office space and offer them a safe, germ-free environment if they bunker down and stay there 24/7. Assign rotating shifts so you have 24 hour presence of people to act as guards. Make sure that they are emotionally stable, rational, trained in security and not afraid to use force to protect the business from outside threats. Plan for the future. The pandemic will abate sooner or later. When you are finally are able to go outside again, you might find your neighbouring and competing businesses looted, abandoned or burned. You know that your business will have survived, and although you will be facing enormous changes, things will never again be the way they were before. But in a different way, they may be even better.

The High Severity scenario

This is the 'gulp' scenario. The unthinkable. It is the least likely pandemic scenario but the most fearful. It is the wipeout of a tenth of humanity and the guaranteed collapse of law and order everywhere in the world. Gangs will be running rampant, looting and killing. The cities will become uninhabitable. It's feasible that another 500 million to a billion people will die from starvation, crime and other diseases. The house in the country plan that works for Low and Medium is pointless in the High scenario. You can bet that the lawlessness will reach every corner of the country.

Any well-established house will be a target for the roaming crazies. You need to find a location that is as hidden and far away from humanity as possible. If it's just an old fishing lodge or a shed or a treehouse, so be it. You're not going to be comfortable, but you will survive.

If you see the pandemic heading for these levels and the airlines are still flying, you may want to leave your home country altogether. I suggest places where there is very low population density and plenty of water. Some suggestions include Australia's Cape York Peninsula and the coastal Northern Territory, New Zealand's lower South Island and Canada's north-central British Columbia. These are currently stable, low-population density countries with decent law-abiding people and are less likely than most other low-density countries, such as Russia to fall completely into chaos. If you're entering another country, don't worry about your visa, just enter as a tourist as the governments will soon break down and then Immigration is certainly not going to come looking for you.

Don't take much cash with you, just enough to get there. It may be worthless soon enough. Have something with you of great value that is small, light and can be traded. Gold and platinum may be worth nothing. Antiviral or vaccine may be worth months of food per course, and they are very light and easy to transport. A bag of Tamiflu might be worth much more than a bag of diamonds.

Due to the fact that this scenario calls for at least two subsequent pandemic waves lasting well over a year it becomes impractical if not downright impossible to stock up on sufficient food and water. Check the survivalist books and websites. Learn to live off the land, what is edible and what is not. Get over your squeamishness and hunt everything that moves. Never touch your prey without rubber gloves and cook it until it's charred.

Even if you're not religious, pick a deity and pray that it will all be over soon.

A bluebird ending

The term 'bluebird ending' was once used to describe a particular penchant of Hollywood studios where they would shoot two endings for some movies. The dramatic, gritty ending would be used for European releases as the studio moguls felt that the continental audiences were more accustomed to realism and tragedy. In these endings, the lovely heroine often succumbed to some dastardly deed or illness and the strapping young hero fell into despair or suicide. However, for the American release, they would splice in some often highly improbable 'happy ending' where the hero and heroine magically overcame all the conflicts in a minute or two of screen time and settled down in the final reel to live happily ever after in a little suburban cottage with a white picket fence. This policy of 'happy endings' at any cost found its greatest expression in the famous studio boss' exclamation: 'No way . . . the kids gotta live at the end of the picture' in *Romeo and Juliet*.

I'm giving you the option of choosing your own ending to this book. You can choose the grim, apocalyptic vision of a ravaged planet, cemeteries overflowing with bodies, and a global economy so ravaged that it will never recover. Or you can choose the ending that H5N1 will take an unpredictable deviation and become a strictly animal flu not generally transmissible to humans, thus the large-scale pandemic will never surface.

Will the human race fall into despair or live happily ever after at the end of the picture? Only time will tell.

Resources

The companies shown in this Resources Guide are not necessarily the only retailers or wholesalers of the products shown. No representations, endorsements or warranties for expected usage are made. Subject to change without notice.

Chapter 5

Female Urinary Aids

EeZeeWee
14 Rust & Vrede Business Square, 21 Church Street,
Durbanville, 7550, South Africa
Tel: +27-21-975-1170, Fax: +27-21-975-2108
Web: www.mouldmed.co.za, Email: gerrit@mouldmed.co.za

Whizzy4You
New Angle Products
Box 25641, Chicago, Illinois 60625, US
Tel: +1-773-478-6779, Fax: Not available
Web: whizzy4you.com, Email: whizzy4you@aol.com

Alcohol Hand Sanitisers

Excalibur Chemicals
40 Baldwin Way, Swindon, Dudley DY3 4PF, UK
Tel: 01384-400690, Fax: 01384-402223
Web: mikeexcal@aol.com, Email: www.excalibur-hygiene.co.uk

Resources

Merlin Chemicals
Unit 5 Passfield Business Park, Passfield, Liphook, Hampshire
GU30 7RR, UK
Tel: 01428-751122, Fax: 01428-751133
Web: merlinchemicals.co.uk, Email: sales@merlinchemicals.co.uk

Medisave (UK)
Units A, B and F McKay Way, Lynch Lane Industrial Estate,
Weymouth, Dorset DT4 9DN, UK
Tel: 01305-784447, Fax: 01305-783583
Web: www.medisave.co.uk, Email: Form on website

Elixir Body Care
3 Tolley Court, Hope Valley SA 5090, Australia
Tel: 08-8263-4144, Fax: 08-8263-4188
Web: www.elixirbodycare.com.au, Email: Form on website

Daylabels
28–32 George Street, Sandringham Victoria 3191, Australia
Tel: 03-9598-8988, Fax: 03-9598-7949
Web: www.daydots.com.au, Email: Form on website

DuPont Virkon S

This product is widely available in agricultural and farm supply retailers.

DuPont Animal Health Solutions
Chilton Industrial Estate, Sudbury, Suffolk CO10 2XD, UK
Tel: 01787-377305, Fax: 01787-310846
Web: www.antecint.com, E-mail: biosecurity@gbr.dupont.com

DuPont (Australia) Ltd
Head Office, 168 Walker Street, North Sydney NSW 2060,
Australia
Tel: 02-9923-6111, Fax: 02-9923-6011
Web: www.au.dupont.com, Email: Form on website

Spa and Hot Tub Chemicals

Swimmingpool Chemicals
Unit 5 Pool Bank Business Park, High Street, Tarvin, Chester
CH3 8JH, UK

Tel: 08003-586140, Fax: Not Available
Web: www.swimmingpoolchemicals.co.uk,
Email: sales@swimmingpoolchemicals.co.uk

The Hot Tub Shop
Brownlow Centre, Lincoln Road, Faldingworth, Lincs LN8 3SF, UK
Tel: 01673-885333, Fax: 01673-885235
Web: www.thehottubshop.co.uk,
Email: shop@thehottubshop.co.uk

The Spa Showrooms
2 East Court, South Bristol Trade Park, Winterstoke Road, Bristol BS3 2LD, UK
Tel: 0117-934-1670, Fax: Not available
Web: www.hotspring.co.uk, Email: bristol@hotspring.co.uk

Spa Parts
4 Salem Court, Lammermoor Beach QLD 4703, Australia
Tel: 07-4933-7744, Fax: 07-4933-7799
Web: www.spaparts.com.au, Email: info@spaparts.com.au

Pool Systems Pty Ltd
79 Kremzow Road, Brendale QLD 4500, Australia
Tel: 07-3889-6722, Fax: 07-3889-6614
Web: www.poolsystems.com.au,
Email: sales@poolsystems.com.au

The Spa Doctor
Box Hill South, Vic 3121, Australia
Tel: 03-9877-1110, Fax: 04-2193-4227
Web: www.thespadoctor.com.au, Email: Form on website

Classic Duo 750 Dishwasher

Akro Foodservice Equipment
16 Blackberry Way, Red Lodge, Suffolk IP28 8TE, UK
Tel: 08701-904091, Fax: 08701-904095
Web: www.akroservices.co.uk, Email: sales@akroservices.co.uk

K.B. Catering
Unit 15 Craven Way, Newmarket, Suffolk CB8 0BW, UK

Tel: 01638-667994, Fax: 01638-665970
Web: www.kb-catering.co.uk, Email: sales@kb-catering.co.uk

CE Online
81 Teme Street, Tenbury Wells, Worcs WR15 8AE, UK
Tel: 08702-402074, Fax: 08702-414-209
Web: www.ceonline.co.uk, Email: info@ceonline.co.uk

Commercial High Temp Dishwashers

Sydney Commercial Kitchens
PO Box 6103 DC, Frenchs Forest NSW 2086, Australia
Tel: 02-9972-0075, Fax: 02-9984-1958
Web: www.sydneycommercialkitchens.com.au,
Email: info@sydneycommercialkitchens.com.au

CDS Commercial Dishwashers
6 Clarke Way, Bassendean WA 6054, Australia
Tel: 08-9377-2036, Fax: Not available
Web: None

N, R and P Respirators

Cole-Parmer Instrument
Unit 3 River Brent Business Park, Trumpers Way, Hanwell,
London W7 2QA, UK
Tel: 020-8574-7556, Fax: 020-8574-7543
Web: www.coleparmer.co.uk, Email: sales@coleparmer.co.uk

Altec Products
Bude Business Centre, Bude, Cornwall EX23 8QN, UK
Tel: 01288-357820, Fax: 01288-357822
Web: www.altecweb.com, Email:sales@altecweb.com

UK Survive
Marlborough House, 37 Prospect Hill, Redditch, Worcs B97
4BS, UK
Tel: 01527-60800, Fax: 01527-61121
Web: www.uksurvive.com, Email: Form on website

Surgical Face Masks
30 Duke Street, Windsor, Berks SL4 7SA, UK
Tel: 01628-777007, Fax: Not available

Web: www.surgical-face-masks.co.uk
Email: sales@surgical-face-masks.co.uk

Bacou-Dalloz
3 Walker Street, Braeside, Vic 3195, Australia
Tel: 03-9587-1500, Fax: 03-9580-8101
Web: www.bacou-dalloz.com, Email: Form on website

Cardinal Health 200 Pty Ltd
Address not available
Tel: 02-9830-0111, Fax: 02-9830-0130
Web: www.cardinalhealth.com.au,
Email: au.customers@cardinal.com

Nanomask

Emergency Filtration Products
175 Cassia Way, Henderson, Nevada 89014, US
Tel: +1-702-558-5164, Fax: +1-702-567-1893
Web: www.emergencyfiltration.com, Email: Not available

UV Portable Handheld

*Ultraviolet light can be extremely hazardous to skin and eyes.
Always wear protective clothing and goggles and never use
ultraviolet light products contrary to manufacturer's instructions.*

UVItec
Avebury House, 36a Union Lane, Cambridge CB4 1QB, UK
Tel: 01223-568060, Fax: 01223-306198
Web: www.uvitec.co.uk, Email: matt@uvitec.co.uk

UV Light Technology
The Light House, 582–584 Hagley Road West, Birmingham
B68 0BS, UK
Tel: 01214-232000, Fax: 01214-232050
Web: www.uv-light.co.uk, Email: sales@uv-light.co.uk

Wolf Laboratories
Wolf House, 80 Market Street, Pocklington, York YO42 2AB,
UK
Tel: 01759-301142, Fax: 01759-301143
Web: www.wolflabs.co.uk, Email: sales@wolflabs.co.uk

Resources

SDR Clinical Technology
213 Eastern Valley Way, Middle Cove, NSW 2068, Australia
Tel: 02-9958-2688, Fax: 02-9958-2655
Web: www.sdr.com.au, Email sdr@sdr.com.au

Extech
2 Langwith Avenue, Boronia, Vic 3155, Australia
Tel: 03-9761-3300, Fax: None
Web: www.extech.com.au, Email: extech@extech.com.au

UV Lamps

*Ultraviolet light can be extremely hazardous to skin and eyes.
Always wear protective clothing and goggles and never use
ultraviolet light products contrary to manufacturer's instructions.*

Ultra-Violet Products
Unit 1 Trinity Hall Farm Estate, Nuffield Road, Cambridge
CB4 1TG, UK
Tel: 01223-420022, Fax: 01223-420561
Web: www.uvp.co.uk, Email: uvp@uvp.co.uk

CP Lighting
Unit 25 Red Lion Road Business Centre, Red Lion Road,
Surbiton, Surrey KT6 7QD, UK
Tel: 020-8391-7474, Fax: 020-8391-7475
Web: www.cp-lighting.co.uk,
Email: sales@cp-lighting.co.uk

AGPC Hygiene
Keeper's Corner, Kennylands Road, Sonning Common,
Reading, Berks RG4 9JP, UK
Tel: 01189-724895, Fax: 01189-724518
Web: www.hygieneshop.co.uk,
Email: mail@hygieneshop.co.uk

Warsash Scientific
Unit 7, The Watertower, 1 Marian Street, Redfern NSW 2016,
Australia
Tel: +61 2 9319 0122, Fax: +61 2 9318 2192
Web: www.warsash.com.au,
Email: sales@warsash.com.au

Beat the Flu

Kelly Company Pty Ltd,
208 Walters Road, Arndell Park, Sydney NSW 2148, Australia
Tel: 02-9672-1500, Fax: 02-9672-1633
Web: None, Email: kellycompany@bigpond.com

PathTech Pty Ltd,
46 Swanston Street, Preston, VIC 3072, Australia
Tel: 03-8480-3500, Fax: 03-8480-3555
Web: www.pathtech.com.au,
Email: customer.service@pathtech.com.au

UVGI Upper Room

Ultraviolet light can be extremely hazardous to skin and eyes. Always wear protective clothing and goggles and never use ultraviolet light products contrary to manufacturer's instructions.

Commercial Lamp Supplies
Unit 2 Revill Court, The Airport Business Park, Exeter EX5 2UL, UK
Tel: 01392-446666, Fax: 01392-447777
Web: www.commercial-lamps.co.uk,
Email: sales@commercial-lamps.co.uk

UVGI Systems
Unit 14 Sherrington Way, Basingstoke RG22 4DQ, UK
Tel: 01256-330479, Fax: 01256-819781
Web: www.diffusion-group.co.uk,
Email: sueb@diffusion-at.co.uk

Suvair
77 Upper Trinity Street, Birmingham B9 4EG, UK
Tel: 01217-712985, Fax: 01217-733004
Web: www.suvair.com, Email: Not available

AES Environmental Pty Ltd
18 Byrne Street, Auburn, NSW 2144, Australia
Tel: 02-8737-8200, Fax: 02-8737-8100
Web: www.aesenvironmental.com.au,
Email: Form on website

Resources

Heraeus
Unit 4, 41–49 Norcal Road, Nunawading, Victoria, 3131,
Australia
Tel: 03-9874-7455, Fax: 03-9874-7488
Web: www.heraeus-amba.com.au,
Email: admin@heraeus-amba.com.au

UV Air Purifiers

*Ultraviolet light can be extremely hazardous to skin and eyes.
Never look inside a UV Air Purifier or use contrary to manufacturer's instructions.*

Zetacool
416–418 London Road, Isleworth, Middlesex TW7 5XB, UK
Tel: 08454-500050, Fax: 020-8568-7194
Web: www.zetacool.com, Email: sales@zetacool.com

Clean Environment Technology
Unit 6 Jubilee Trading Estate, Newcastle Road, Congleton,
Cheshire CW12 4SB, UK
Tel: 01260-297722, Fax: 01260-297744
Web: www.bioair.co.uk, Email: Form on website

Air Purification Systems
208 Chester Road, Warrington, Cheshire WA4 6AR, UK
Tel: 01925-242606, Fax: 01925-242088
Web: www.airpurificationsystems.co.uk,
E-mail: admin@airpurificationsystems.co.uk

Airiononics
Level 1, Suite 18, Greenview Corporate Centre, 20
Commercial Road, Melbourne, Victoria 3004, Australia
Tel: 03-9820-4022, Fax: 03-9867-4033
Web: www.airiononics.com.au,
Email: iononics@dragon.net.au

Cardiffair Control Systems Pty Ltd
1210 Logan Road, PO BOX 30, Holland Park QLD 4121,
Australia
Tel: 07-3343-7499, Fax: 07-3343-7599
Web: www.cardiffair.com.au, Email: sales@cardiffair.com.au

Sharp Plasmacluster

The Healthy House
The Old Co-op, Lower Street, Ruscombe, Stroud,
Gloucestershire GL6 6BU, UK
Tel: 01453-752216, Fax: 01453-753533
Web: www.healthy-house.co.uk,
Email: info@healthy-house.co.uk

Sharp Electronics (UK)
Sharp House, Thorp Road, Manchester M40 5BE, UK
Tel: 0161-2052333, Fax: 0161-2057076
Web: www.sharp.co.uk, Email: Form on website

Electrical Discount UK
81 Northgate, Blackburn, Lancashire BB2 1AA, UK
Tel: 01282-818472, Fax: 01282-818451
Web: www.electricaldiscountuk.co.uk,
Email: enquiries@electricaldiscountuk.co.uk

Curry's Superstores
Locations throughout the UK
Tel: 08701-545570, Fax: Not available
Web: www.currys.co.uk,
Email: customer.services@currys.co.uk

Halas Supply
Unit 1, 44 O'Dea Avenue, Waterloo NSW 2017, Locked Bag
No. 5003, Alexandria NSW 2015, Australia
Tel: 02-9697-6288, Fax: 02-9697-6250
Web: www.halas.com.au, Email: info@halas.com.au

Shire Air Conditioning
PO Box 900, Sutherland NSW 1499, Australia
Tel: 02-9548-3444, Fax: 02-9548-1123
Web: www.shireair.com.au, Email: sales@shireair.com.au

Sharp Corporation of Australia
1 Huntingwood Drive, Blacktown NSW 2148, Australia
Tel: 1300-135022, Fax: 1300-727717
Web: www.sharp.net.au,
Email: Form on website

Resources

Smaller-fitting condoms

Sensible Johnny
22 Brassmill Enterprise Centre, Brassmill Lane, Bath,
Somerset BA1 3JN, UK
Tel: 08009-156635, Fax: Not available
Web: www.sensiblejohnny.co.uk,
Email: customercare@sensiblejohnny.co.uk

Condoms Direct
28 Ashleigh Meadows, Rathfriland, Newry BT34 5RN, UK
Tel: 08452-262697, Fax: Not available
Web: www.condoms-direct.com,
Email: sales@condoms-direct.com

Big Boy Ltd
Castle View, Cleers, Roche, Cornwall PL26 8ND, UK
Tel: Not available, Fax: Not available
Web: www.bigboycondoms.co.uk,
Email: info@bigboycondoms.co.uk

Condoms WebDirect
P.O. Box 123, Chorley, Lancashire PR6 9FD, UK
Tel: 01257-483067, Fax: Not available
Web: www.condoms.co.uk, Email: sales@condoms.co.uk

Condom Country
PO Box 227, Croydon NSW 2132, Australia
Tel: 02-8756-3569, Fax: 02-8756-3577
Web: www.condomcountry.com.au,
Email: orders@condomcountry.com.au

Adult Shop
118 Roe Street, Northbridge WA 6003, Australia
Tel: 08-9227-6777, Fax: 08-9227-6788
Web: www.shop.adultshop.com.au,
Email: ozinfo@adultshop.com

Chapter 7

Goggles

Simon Safety
Unit 73, Honeyborough Industrial Estate, Neyland,
Milford Haven, Pembrokeshire SA73 1SE
Tel: 01646-600750, Fax: 01646-602299
Web: www.simon-safety.co.uk, Email: Form on website

Tooled-Up.com
78 Suez Road, Ponders End
Brimsdown, Enfield, Middlesex, EN3 7PS
Tel: 0870-2408141, Fax: 020-8805-4545
Web: www.tooled-up.com, Email: Form on website

Uvex Safety Australia
PO Box 6144, Parramatta NSW 2150
Tel: 02-9891-1700, Fax: 02-9891-1788
Web: www.uvex.com.au, Email: info@uvex.com.au

B Protected
Unit 5, 147 Foster Street, Dandenong, Melbourne, Victoria 3175
Tel: 03-9792-1380, Fax: 03-9706-8867
Web: www.b-protected.com.au

Chapter 8

Propolis, zinc lozenges, and Vitamin C are readily available at various retailers in your area. The best way to find these companies in your area is to consult your local Yellow Page directory or online listings for Health Foods, Alternative or Complementary Health and Therapies. Many of the other products are available in any supermarket or pharmacy. Colloidal silver is available from the retailers listed in Chapter 5 under Spa and Hot Tub Chemicals, however it is strictly not advised to take colloidal silver internally. Cannabis is also widely available in your area but also strictly not recommended. The rest of the products you'd be crazy to use anyway, so you can source them yourself.

Resources

Chapter 9

Most of the world's online pharmaceutical supply comes from Canada and they usually are the best choice to have rare antivirals in stock. These online pharmacies were asked to quote on various quantities of Tamiflu 75-milligram tablets. They are listed from least expensive to most expensive, excluding shipping and other charges. As in the rest of this book, the currency exchange rates were accurate at the time of writing. These online pharmacies are members of leading industry associations, thus are among the most reputable suppliers in this random sampling. Some telephone numbers listed may be difficult to reach from outside the US or Canada as they are toll-free in North America. Check with your long distance telephone provider for access and costs.

adv-care.com
Hours of Operation: Monday to Friday, 9.00 am to 6.00 pm, Eastern Standard Time (GMT-4)
CEO/President: Not Listed
70 Esna Park Drive, Markham, Ontario L3R 6E7, Canada
Pharmacist Manager: M Bannis
Email: pharmacist@adv-care.com
Tel: +1-888-471-4721 Customer Service/General Information
Email: service@adv-care.com
Tel: +1-888-471-4721, Fax: +1-877-948-0464
Affiliated Physical Pharmacy(ies):
Adv Care Pharmacy
Licensed by: Florida Board of Pharmacy PH19692, US
AdvCare Pharmacy, Inc.
Licensed by: Ontario College of Pharmacists Accreditation #038132, Canada
Quoted cost in September 2005 of Tamiflu 10-pack £26.94/$48.49

canadadrugs.com
Hours of Operation: Customer Service: Monday to Sunday, 24 Hours/day. Pharmacy: Monday to Friday, 7.30 am to 11.30 pm, Saturday and Sunday, 8.00 am to 6.00 pm, Central Standard Time (GMT-5)

Beat the Flu

CEO/President: Kris Thorkelson
24 Terracon Place, Winnipeg, Manitoba R2J 4G7, Canada
Pharmacist Manager: Robert Fraser
Email: pharmacist@canadadrugs.com
Tel +1-800-226-3784
Customer Service/General Information
Email: info@canadadrugs.com
Tel: +1-800-226-3784, Fax: +1-877-525-8539
Affiliated Physical Pharmacy(ies)
CanadaDrugs.com
Licensed by: Manitoba Pharmaceutical Association – Licence #32195, Canada
Quoted cost in September 2005 of Tamiflu: 10-pack £27.26/$49.07, 20-pack: £54.51/$98.12

rxnorth.com
Hours of Operation: Monday to Friday, 7.00 am to 9.00 pm, Saturday, 8.00 am to 4.00 pm, Central Standard Time (GMT-5)
CEO/President: Andrew Strempler
115 Main St. South, Minnedosa, Manitoba R0J 1EO, Canada
Pharmacist Manager: Andrew Strempler
Email: generalinfo@rxnorth.com
Tel: +1-888-773-2698
Customer Service/General Information
Email: generalinfo@rxnorth.com
Tel: +1-888-773-2698, Fax: +1-888-773-2696
Affiliated Physical Pharmacy(ies)
Mediplan Pharmacy
Licensed by: Manitoba Pharmaceutical Association – Licence #31958, Canada
Quoted cost in September 2005 of Tamiflu 10-pack £29.71/$53.48

pharmacy-online.ca
Hours of Operation: Monday to Friday, 9.00 am to 9.00 pm, Saturday, 9.00 am to 3.00 pm, Mountain Standard Time (GMT-6)
CEO/President: Barney Briton
#500, 400 Crowfoot Crescent NW, Calgary, Alberta T3G 5H6, Canada

Resources

Pharmacist Manager: M Savage
Email: msavage@pharmacy-online.ca
Tel: +1-403-693-3110
Customer Service/General Information
Email: general@pharmacy-online.ca
Tel: +1-877-530-3743, Fax: +1-866-540-4110
Affiliated Physical Pharmacy(ies):
Minit Drugs
Licensed by: Alberta College of Pharmacists, Licence #1657,
Canada
*Quoted cost in September 2005 of Tamiflu: 10-pack
£31.11/$56, 20-pack £53.91/$97.04, 50-pack: £122.29/$220.12*

crossborderpharmacy.com
Hours of Operation: Monday to Friday, 6.00 am to 9.00 pm,
Saturday, 8.00 am to 4.00 pm, Mountain Standard Time (GMT-6)
CEO/President: Dave Robertson
Suite 100, 8 Manning Close, Calgary, Alberta T2E 7N5, Canada
Pharmacist Manager: Brent Grantham
Email: pharmacist@crossborderpharmacy.com
Tel: +1-888-626-0696
Customer Service/General Information
Email: info@crossborderpharmacy.com
Tel: +1-888-626-0696, Fax: +1-888-635-0535
Affiliated Physical Pharmacy(ies)
Total Care Pharmacy
Licensed by: Alberta College of Pharmacists – Licence #1537,
Canada
*Quoted cost in September 2005 of Tamiflu 10-pack:
£29.02/$52.24, 20-pack: £53.26/$95.87, 50-pack:
£125.98/$226.76, 90-pack: £222.94/$401.29*

*The online pharmacies above will also provide Relenza,
Symmetrel and Flumadine, if they have those drugs in
inventory at the time of your contact.*

*The following is a listing of some of the reputable online
pharmacy associations and accreditation boards, followed by
the website addresses of the online pharmacies that were
members in good standing as of September 2005. Any of these*

*online pharmacies may provide Tamiflu, Relenza, Symmetrel
and Flumadine if they are available. Each has a different policy on doctor's prescription requirements prior to selling drugs
internationally. Some may require a hard copy, some others a
fax, some others a self-evaluation and some others may
require no prescription or self-qualification at all. Contact
them for their policies. Contact information is listed on each
of their websites. All of the following website addresses
should be prefixed with* http://www *in your browser. No representations are made for any of these associations or their
member online pharmacies.*

Canadian International Pharmacy Association
Krys Kirton, Executive Assistant
521–70 Arthur Street, Winnipeg, Manitoba R3B 1G7, Canada
Tel: +1-204943-7912, Fax: +1-204-943-7926
Web: ciparx.ca,
Email: krys.kirton@ciparx.ca
Member Online Pharmacies: adv-care.com, canadadrugs.com,
canadadrugsonline.com, canadaeastpharmacy.com,
canadamedici neshop.com, canadapharmacy.com,
canadaprescriptionplus.com, canadauspharmacy.com,
canadawaydrugs.com, canadianusapre scriptions.com,
candrug.com, candrugstore.com, doctorsolve.com,
extendedcarepharmacy.com, hometownmeds.com,
ktel drugmart.com, mcgregorclinic.com, medcentercanada.com,
medicationscanada.com, medimartpharmacy.com, medisave.ca,
meds4mail.com, medsforamerica.com, northlandmeds.com, ocu-
source.com, oneworldrx.com, onlinecanadianpharmacy.com,
onlinepharmaciescanada.com, pharmacyincanada.com,
pharmacy-online.ca, rx1.biz, rxcanadiansavings.com, rxnorth.com,
saveoncanadianmeds.com, smartchoicepharmacy.com,
thecanadapharmacy.com, universaldrugstore.com

Impac
Dana Noble, Executive Officer for Operations
P.O. Box 1146, Manchester, Vermont 05254, US
Tel: +1-800-677-7019
Web: impacsurvey.org, Email: Form on website

Resources

Member Online Pharmacies: canadadrugs.com,
canadauspharmacy.com, canadiandrugstore.com,
crossborderpharmacy.com, kteldrugmart.com,
pharmacy-online.ca, rxnorth.com, swiftrx.com

Pharmacy Checker
Tod Cooperman, President
333 Mamaroneck Avenue, White Plains, New York 10605, US
Phone: +718-387-4526, Fax: +718-715-1033
Web: pharmacychecker.com
Email: info@pharmacychecker.com
Member Online Pharmacies: adv-care.com, affordablerx.com,
canadadiscountrx.com, canadadrugs.com, canadameds.com,
canadarxpharmacy.com, canadauspharmacy.com,
canadiandrugs.ca, clickmeds.com, costco.com,
crossborderpharmacy.com, cvs.com, doctorsolve.com,
globalcanadarx.com, globalchemist.com, jandrugs.com,
kwikmed.com, lifhaus.ca, magendavidmeds.com,
medicationscanada.com, meds4mail.com, medsmex.com,
northlandmeds.com, onlinecanadianpharmacy.com,
pharmacy-online.ca, planetdrugsdirect.com,
prescriptionpoint.com, rxcarecanada.com, rxinternational.com,
rxnorth.com, thecanadiandrugstore.com,
thecanadianpharmacy.com, ukmedsdirect.com,
universaldrugstore.com, valuepharmaceuticals.com

Some of the major Australian online pharmacies include:
epharmacy.com.au
onlinepharmacy.com.au
emedical.com.au
jumbopharmacy.com.au

*You may be well advised to contact your local Pharmaceutical
Boards for further information on the policy and restrictions of
purchasing and importing Tamiflu, Relenza, Symmetrel and/or
Flumadine:*

Royal Pharmaceutical Society of Great Britain
Ann M Lewis, Secretary and Registrar
1 Lambeth High Street, London SE1 7JN, UK

Tel: 020-7735-9141, Fax: 020-7735-7629
Email: enquiries@rpsgb.org, Web: rpsgb.org.uk

Scottish Department
36 York Place, Edinburgh, EH1 3HU, UK
Tel: 0131-5564386, Fax: 0131-5588850
Email: info@rpsis.com

Welsh Executive
Gloucester House, 14 Mount Stuart Square, Cardiff
CF10 5DP, UK
Tel: 02920-412800, Fax: 02920-412810
Email: wales@rpsgb.org

ACT Pharmacy Board: healthregboards.act.gov.au
Pharmaceutical Council of Western Australia: pcwa.com.au
Pharmacists Board of Queensland: pharmacyboard.qld.gov.au
Pharmacy Board of New South Wales: phbnsw.org.au
Pharmacy Board of South Australia: pharmacyboard.sa.gov.au
Pharmacy Board of Tasmania: regboardstas.com/pharmacy
Pharmacy Board of Victoria: pharmacybd.vic.gov.au

Chapter 12

UK
Personal finance advice is an enormous industry in both the UK and Australia and there are hundreds of financial advisers in every region of both countries.

In the UK, the Personal Finance Society is the largest professional body for individual financial advisers (and those in related roles):
The Personal Finance Society
20 Aldermanbury, London EC2V 7HY, UK
Tel: 020-8530852, Fax: 020-7796- 3882
Web: www.thepfs.org, Email: customer.serv@thepfs.org

In Australia the only national financial planning professional body is the FPA:

Resources

Financial Planning Association of Australia Limited
PO Box 234, Collins Street West, Melbourne, VIC 8007,
Australia
Tel: 03-9614-2289, Fax: 03-9614-1912
Web: www.fpa.asn.au, Email: fpa@fpa.asn.au

Chapter 13

Air filters and purifiers: See Chapter 5 Resources

Alcohol hand sanitisers: See Chapter 5 Resources

Antiviral: See Chapter 9 Resources

Batteries: Check your local Yellow Page directory for
Wholesale Electrical and Electronics

Bleach: Check your local Yellow Page directory for Wholesale
Janitorial Supplies

Bottled water: Check your local Yellow Page directory for
Wholesale Water Suppliers

Camp stoves: Check your local Yellow Page directory for
Wholesale Camping and Outdoor Equipment

Candles: Check your local Yellow Page directory for
Wholesale Candles

Dried, canned and jarred food: Check your local Yellow Page
directory for Wholesale Foods

Electric generators: Check your local Yellow Page directory
for Wholesale Generators

First aid kits: Check your local Yellow Page directory for
Wholesale First Aid Supplies

Folk flu remedies: See Chapter 8 Resources

Fuel of any kind: Check your local Yellow Page directory for
Wholesale Fuel Distributors

Funeral and morgue supplies: Check your local Yellow Page directory for Wholesale Funeral Supplies

Goggles: Check your local Yellow Page directory for Wholesale Industrial Safety Equipment

Heat pads: Check your local Yellow Page directory for Wholesale Camping and Outdoor Equipment

Hydrogen peroxide: Check your local Yellow Page directory for Wholesale Pharmacy Supplies

Inhalers: Check your local Yellow Page directory for Wholesale Pharmacy Supplies

Respirators: See Chapter 5 Resources

Rubber gloves: Check your local Yellow Page directory for Wholesale Janitorial Supplies

Rubbing alcohol: Check your local Yellow Page directory for Wholesale Pharmacy Supplies

Stay-dry matches: Check your local Yellow Page directory for Wholesale Camping and Outdoor Supplies

Survivalist and camping gear: Check your local Yellow Page directory for Wholesale Camping and Outdoor Supplies

Water filters and purifiers: Check your local Yellow Page directory for Wholesale Water Treatment

Wind-up radios: Check your local Yellow Page directory for Wholesale Camping and Outdoor Supplies

Acknowledgements

Special mention must be made here of a few individuals: Dr Mike Skinner, for his invaluable input and contribution, Dr Henry Niman, for his hourly updates on the state of the virus, and Robin and Liz Puttick and all the folks at Fusion Press, for believing in an H5N1 book months before the media hysteria began.

About the Author

A A Avlicino is a 48-year-old Italian-Canadian medical researcher and science writer living in rural Dorset, England. His published Dialylitic Retroviral Treatment paper was presented at the 1994 AIDS Conference, Yokohama, Japan. He conducted an HIV Epidemiological Study in conjunction with the AIDS Action Group, Tampa Bay, Florida, US. He developed an ultraviolet light emitter for viral/bacterial disinfection in hospitals.

As Editor and Associate Publisher he was responsible for a total of 25 magazines and scientific/medical journal titles, including *Kyklosian*, a wholistic science journal, and *Whale & Dolphin*, a cetacean biology journal, and wrote hundreds of articles for these periodicals. He has been a member of the Canadian Society for Medical Laboratory Science and has presented his varied research findings at international conferences at universities in Europe, US, Australia and Japan.